PRESCRIPTION (Rx) for Parenting

How to Raise Healthy Infants and Children

Charlotte E. Thompson, M.D.

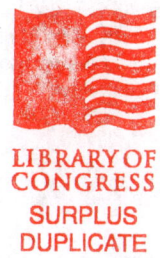

Prescription (Rx) for Parenting:
How to Raise Healthy Infants and Children

Copyright © 2015 by Atlantic Publishing Group, Inc.
1405 SW 6th Ave. • Ocala, Florida 34471 • 800-814-1132 • 352-622-1875–Fax
Website: www.atlantic-pub.com • E-mail: sales@atlantic-pub.com
SAN Number: 268-1250

No part of this publication may be reproduced, stored in a retrieval system, or transmitted in any form or by any means, electronic, mechanical, photocopying, recording, scanning, or otherwise, except as permitted under Section 107 or 108 of the 1976 United States Copyright Act, without the prior written permission of the Publisher. Requests to the Publisher for permission should be sent to Atlantic Publishing Group, Inc., 1405 SW 6th Ave., Ocala, Florida 34471.

Library of Congress Cataloging-in-Publication Data

Thompson, Charlotte E.
  Prescription (Rx) for parenting : how to raise healthy infants and children / by Charlotte E. Thompson, M.D.
       pages cm
  ISBN 978-1-62023-036-7 (alk. paper) -- ISBN 1-62023-036-4 (alk. paper) 1. Parenting. 2. Children--Health and hygiene. 3. Child rearing. I. Title.
  HQ755.8.T563 2015
  649'.1--dc23
                              2015005004

LIMIT OF LIABILITY/DISCLAIMER OF WARRANTY: The publisher and the author make no representations or warranties with respect to the accuracy or completeness of the contents of this work and specifically disclaim all warranties, including without limitation warranties of fitness for a particular purpose. No warranty may be created or extended by sales or promotional materials. The advice and strategies contained herein may not be suitable for every situation. This work is sold with the understanding that the publisher is not engaged in rendering legal, accounting, or other professional services. If professional assistance is required, the services of a competent professional should be sought. Neither the publisher nor the author shall be liable for damages arising herefrom. The fact that an organization or website is referred to in this work as a citation and/or a potential source of further information does not mean that the author or the publisher endorses the information the organization or website may provide or recommendations it may make. Further, readers should be aware that Internet websites listed in this work may have changed or disappeared between when this work was written and when it is read.

TRADEMARK: All trademarks, trade names, or logos mentioned or used are the property of their respective owners and are used only to directly describe the products being provided. Every effort has been made to properly capitalize, punctuate, identify and attribute trademarks and trade names to their respective owners, including the use of ® and ™ wherever possible and practical. Atlantic Publishing Group, Inc. is not a partner, affiliate, or licensee with the holders of said trademarks.

Printed in the United States

Printed on Recycled Paper

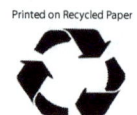

Reduce. Reuse. RECYCLE.

A decade ago, Atlantic Publishing signed the Green Press Initiative. These guidelines promote environmentally friendly practices, such as using recycled stock and vegetable-based inks, avoiding waste, choosing energy-efficient resources, and promoting a no-pulping policy. We now use 100-percent recycled stock on all our books. The results: in one year, switching to post-consumer recycled stock saved 24 mature trees, 5,000 gallons of water, the equivalent of the total energy used for one home in a year, and the equivalent of the greenhouse gases from one car driven for a year.

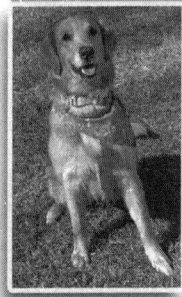 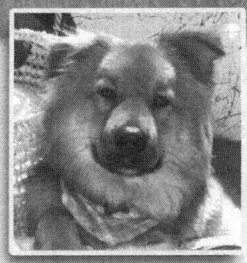 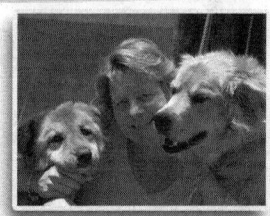

Over the years, we have adopted a number of dogs from rescues and shelters. First there was Bear and after he passed, Ginger and Scout. Now, we have Kira, another rescue. They have brought immense joy and love not just into our lives, but into the lives of all who met them.

We want you to know a portion of the profits of this book will be donated in Bear, Ginger and Scout's memory to local animal shelters, parks, conservation organizations, and other individuals and nonprofit organizations in need of assistance.

– ***Douglas & Sherri Brown,***
President & Vice-President of Atlantic Publishing

In Memory
of
My Daughter, Jennifer
Who is So Greatly Missed

Table of Contents

Foreword *6*

Introduction *7*

Section 1 Rx for Babies and Infants *8*

Section 2 Rx for Toddler Behavior Problems *48*

Section 3 Rx for Parenting PreSchoolers *85*

Section 4 Rx for Parenting Kids *110*

Resources *147*

Bibliography *153*

Index *155*

Foreword

Dr. Charlotte E. Thompson has written a book that will serve as a much-needed guide to all those who have the pleasure of working with young children. Dozens of useful suggestions clearly explain practical advice from a noted pediatrician who has dedicated her life to assisting mothers, fathers, teachers and guardians.

I have had the great pleasure of knowing Dr. Thompson for over 50 years when she became my son's doctor. In turn, our professional relationship grew when I became her son's second grade teacher. Years later her grandchildren attended the independent school where I was the Head.

The sections ahead explain ways to handle so many important questions about babies, toddlers and preschoolers. Dr. Thompson has provided helpful suggestions to address such issues as crying, day care, temper tantrums, discipline, toilet training, independence, and making friends.

Parents and caregivers will find this reference to be useful on a daily basis.

Moreen Fielden
BA, Stanford University
Retired Head of The Gillispie School
La Jolla, California

Introduction

As a young mother, I would have loved to have had a book giving me practical advice about caring for infants and children. I had an M.D. degree from Stanford Medical School and a license to practice medicine, but knew absolutely nothing about the day-to-day care of a newborn or how to raise a child. We were given good pediatric training, but it was mostly about diagnosing and treating sick babies and children. There were classes on child development, but they were no help to me when Jennifer was not sleeping, having difficulty nursing, or crying. The hospital where she was born did not have a nursing consultant and the pediatrician just checked for problems. In many ways, I think this lack of help made me a better pediatrician, because I could understand the fear mothers and fathers feel when confronted with a crying, miserable newborn or child or one who will not sleep or eat.

In a new office, I had a small room added where mothers could nurse their babies and added a classroom and treatment room. I made many house calls, answered my own telephone when I was on call nights and weekends, and always met parents in hospital emergency rooms. In addition, printed sheets were provided about various problems which parents told me were of great help. Some of the advice and instructions have been incorporated into this book, as well as answers to the many questions I was asked by mothers and fathers.

I hope this book will help all readers find the joy in parenting that one father has found. Recently he said to me, "My wife and I have so much fun with our children."

Section 1

BABIES AND INFANTS

Includes Parenting Prescriptions for:

BREAST FEEDING 9	BATHING 30
SLEEPING 10	CLOTHING 31
CRYING 11	TEETHING 32
TIPS FOR MOTHERS 12	BURPING 32
TIPS FOR FATHERS 13	PETS 33
ALLERGIES 14	CHILDPROOFING YOUR HOUSE 34
TRAVELING 15	
SUPPORT 16	INFANTS WITH SPECIAL NEEDS 35
CONSTIPATION 17	INFANT SCHEDULES 36
MEDICAL CONCERNS 18	INFANT CPR 36
SAFETY 19	IMMUNIZATION TIPS 37
DAYCARE 20	GROWING STEPS 38
FINDING AND HIRING CHILDCARE WORKER 21	HAVING FUN 38
	SINGLE PARENTING 39
EATING 22	MOTION 40
EMERGENCIES 23	EQUIPMENT 41
INFORMATION FOR CHILDCARE WORKERS 24	SOUND 42
	COLIC 43
FINDING A DOCTOR 25	SUPPLIES 44
CHOOSING AN HMO OR HEALTH INSURANCE 26	PREMATURE BABIES 45
	SCHEDULES FOR WELL CHECKUPS 46
TWINS/MULTIPLE BIRTHS 27	
TOYS 28	HOSPITALIZATIONS 47
SKIN CARE 29	

BREAST FEEDING

A tired, distraught, young mother with a three-week-old sat in my office with tears welling. The baby was puckering up her face and beginning to cry. "I want so much to nurse Jenny," she said, "but I just don't have enough milk. She cries and cries and I feel like a failure."

"You seem exhausted and need a good night's sleep," I told her. "Can someone else take the baby and give her a bottle? Remember that fatigue and anxiety will decrease the amount of milk you have leaving you with an anxious, fussy baby."

- ✓ Sit in a comfortable chair in a quiet place to nurse.
- ✓ Let others help with shopping and housework.
- ✓ Drink lots of fluids. (Some herbal teas can cause a baby to have diarrhea.)
- ✓ Don't eat spicy foods, garlic, onions, and members of the cabbage family. These can cause tummy aches in babies.
- ✓ Check with your doctor about which drugs pass through breast milk and cause problems.
- ✓ Don't feel guilty if you try hard to nurse and have to stop.
- ✓ Learn to manually express milk in the baby's mouth to start nursing.
- ✓ Start nursing from the alternate breast each time.
- ✓ Use an electric breast pump to express milk if you are going to be away.
- ✓ Don't feel guilty about giving an occasional bottle.

Nursing should be special and not a chore. Don't be pushed into continuing to nurse by a doctor, nurse, friend, family member or the media.

SLEEPING

A mother and grandmother brought in Tommy, a seven-day-old baby, for me to check. Both were tired and upset.

"The baby has kept us all up every night since we brought him home from the hospital," they said. "We've tried everything to help him sleep. Is there anything you can do to help us?" the mother asked. "I had no idea a baby would act like this."

"Let's go over the things you've tried," I said "and then hopefully I'll have some other ideas."

- ✓ Bundle or swaddle a baby in more than one receiving blanket.
- ✓ Use a small cradle or bassinet to help a baby feel snug.
- ✓ In a pinch, a dresser drawer or a big, firm box can be used as a bed.
- ✓ Don't overheat a room as this can make a baby fretful and prevent sleep.
- ✓ Be sure a baby doesn't have a burp that needs to come up.
- ✓ Don't over or under dress a baby because this can interfere with sound sleep.
- ✓ Try motion to help a baby sleep.
- ✓ Have a rocking chair in a baby's room.
- ✓ Put a music box by the bed to help a baby sleep.
- ✓ Go for a car ride. This almost always puts a baby to sleep.
- ✓ Put a baby on his or her back to sleep, not on the face or side.
- ✓ Try rocking a baby to sleep.
- ✓ Don't have a loud TV audible in a baby's room. This can be disturbing.
- ✓ Be sure the baby doesn't have dirty or wet diapers.
- ✓ Try to be relaxed as possible because anxious, tense caretakers can keep babies awake.
- ✓ Be sure a baby isn't hungry.
- ✓ Try giving a baby a pacifier to suck.

SECTION 1: Babies and Infants

CRYING

A new father called one night saying that his infant son seemed colicky and wouldn't stop crying. "I've tried everything that has worked before, but now I am desperate. My wife has gone out to do some errands. I need your help."

I made a few suggestions and then said, "If none of these things work, I would go for a ride in the car."

"With or without the baby, the father asked?" (I think he was serious.)

- ✓ Check for hunger.
- ✓ Check that there are not too few or too many clothes.
- ✓ Check for wet or soiled diapers.
- ✓ Try to get up a burp.
- ✓ Be sure the room isn't too hot or too cold.
- ✓ Be sure the baby's room is quiet and a loud TV or radio can't be heard.
- ✓ Don't have anything dangling near the baby's face.
- ✓ Prevent any excessive stimulation because this can cause a crying, unhappy baby.
- ✓ Try motion to help a baby relax and stop crying.
- ✓ Play soft music or a music box to help stop crying.
- ✓ Don't pick up the baby with each cry. A baby needs to cry from time to time.
- ✓ Give a pacifier to suck.
- ✓ Try giving a little water in a bottle or a pacifier to stop crying.

NOTE: Dr. Barry Brazelton, who followed in Dr. Spock's footsteps as America's number one pediatrician, says babies need to learn to quiet themselves. If they are picked up as soon as they cry, they never learn this ability. Understanding the meaning of each cry usually comes fairly quickly to new parents. There will be a cry for hunger, for a wet or soiled diaper, for pain and for tiredness.

TIPS FOR MOTHERS

A thirty-six-year old first-time mother, who had worked full-time until the birth of her son, brought Jerry in for his first check up. There were dark circles under her eyes and she looked as if she was about to cry.

"I had no idea", she said, "that having a baby would be this difficult. I miss my friends at work so much and can't seem to get anything done during the day. I thought that I was going to have an easy time because I read every book that I could get my hands on and took classes about infant care. PLEASE HELP ME!"

- ✓ Don't lose your individuality. You are still a unique person, not just a mother.
- ✓ Spend at least a few minutes each day to think, plan or just be.
- ✓ Hire some help daily for even an hour or so. This can make a great difference. A teenager or older woman in your neighborhood might be available to help out.
- ✓ Exercise daily or several times a week. This is essential.
- ✓ Plan one morning, afternoon, or evening per week to do exactly what you want.
- ✓ Don't always put a baby or partner's needs ahead of your own. This will create both short-term and long-term physical or emotional problems.
- ✓ Plan weekly time alone with your partner and don't talk about the baby!
- ✓ Connect with other new mothers in a new mothers' group or online in a chat room.
- ✓ Start a new creative project. This can energize and refresh you.
- ✓ Broaden your outlook with art, music, dance, or theater.
- ✓ Join a book group to meet new friends and have adult conversation.

SECTION 1: Babies and Infants (13)

TIPS FOR FATHERS

A new father came to see me because he was so concerned about what was going on at home. He said, "My wife has been distraught, tired, and frazzled since the birth of Ian. I have talked to her obstetrician, but he doesn't seem to hear me. I am willing to take time off from work, get help or do anything that I need to do, but I can only handle so much of the burden. I suspect that my wife is suffering from a mild post-partum depression and am insisting she get some medical help. How do I get though this bad time? I am sure it will get better but for now I need your suggestions."

- ✓ Find a good friend or buddy with whom you can really talk.
- ✓ Get some daily or weekly exercise.
- ✓ Take some weekly time to have fun or just be alone.
- ✓ Find someone to come in and help daily. A teenager or older woman could be a great asset.
- ✓ Join a fathers' group or even go online and chat with other fathers in the same situation.
- ✓ Start a new project or do something entirely different to get your mind off of problems.
- ✓ Plan a weekly date with your wife to do something fun.
- ✓ Treat yourself now and then to a good book, a new CD, or toy.
- ✓ Insist that you and your wife have weekly time together without the baby.
- ✓ Insist on some outside professional help for your wife if she is depressed.
- ✓ Bring your wife an occasional bunch of flowers.
- ✓ Take your turn in caring for the baby. You'll be rewarded in many ways.

ALLERGIES

The parents of a two-month old baby, Jed, whom I had not examined previously, came for a consultation because they were concerned about Jed's loss of weight.

"The baby spits up after each feeding", the mother said. "It isn't just spitting, it's more like vomiting. I tried to nurse him but had problems. Now we have Jed on a bottle." He's also constipated."

"What kind of formula do you have him on?" I asked.

"It's a regular milk formula", the father answered.

After taking a history and examining the baby, I felt that the infant could be allergic since there was a strong family history of allergies. The previous doctor had not suggested that cow's milk could be the problem. By changing the formula to soybean milk, the infant began gaining weight and everyone was happy.

- ✓ Don't forget that a colicky baby may be an allergic baby.
- ✓ Eliminate allergic foods if you are breast-feeding.
- ✓ Don't give or eat foods which can cause problems: chocolate, wheat, nuts, fish, eggs, citrus, cow's milk, and sometimes soybean milk.
- ✓ Start only one new food at a time.
- ✓ Try a new food for a few days before adding something else.
- ✓ Give single foods rather than mixtures.
- ✓ Read the labels on baby food jars.
- ✓ Look for constipation as a sign of wheat intolerance.
- ✓ See a pediatric allergist if there are signs of food intolerance or other allergies.
- ✓ Even small babies can have severe allergies that can show up rather quickly.
- ✓ Look for eczema, which can be a sign of allergy.
- ✓ Get a family history to see if allergies, such as eczema or asthma, are present.
- ✓ Breast-feed, if possible, to delay or prevent the onset of allergies.
- ✓ Try to use non-allergenic soaps, if there is a family history of allergy.
- ✓ Eliminate wool, which can be especially bothersome to a baby with skin problems.
- ✓ Keep a record of frequent stools because this can be a sign of allergy.

TRAVELING

A young navy wife brought Sonja in for her three-week examination. The baby seemed fine, but the mother was tired and upset.

"My husband has been reassigned to a base in Texas", the mother said, "and I'm on my way there now to meet him." "You mean you're leaving today?" I said.

"Yes", she said. "I'm leaving from your office, but I wanted you to check Sonja first."

"Do you have plenty of supplies?" I asked. "Well, I have one bottle", the mother said. "I thought I would pick up things as I needed them along the way. I have been too tired to get much together. "

Fortunately, we had baby samples in the office, so the nurse put diapers, milk, and other things together and we sent the mother on her way. There were tears in her eyes as she left and she couldn't have been more appreciative. I asked the mother to call when she arrived in Texas. She did call three days later, saying all was well. She thanked me again for being sure she traveled with adequate supplies.

- ✓ Make plans before you start on a trip listing everything that might be needed.
- ✓ Take more of everything than you think you'll need.
- ✓ Go through a day, hour by hour, to be sure you anticipate everything you'll need.
- ✓ Carry a small, working flashlight and some extra batteries.
- ✓ Carry lots of Wash n' Dries or Handiwipes in your bag.
- ✓ Have a baby sucking on a pacifier or a bottle during an airplane landing to protect the eardrums.
- ✓ Check with airlines or trains about rules for car seats and strollers prior to your trip.
- ✓ Pack things that you will need as well as the baby's needs. Take along a good book or two and some playing cards.
- ✓ Don't expect flight attendants to help with your baby. They may have their hands full with other tasks.
- ✓ Don't travel when a baby has a cold.
- ✓ Try to keep a small infant away from the other passengers and don't let anyone kiss her or him. They may try!

SUPPORT

A professional mother, who was new to the area, called frantically one night. Her question surprised me because the answer seemed so simple. I knew she had read several baby books and attended infant care classes.

It didn't take me long to discover that the frantic call and subsequent frequent calls were because she had no support system: close friends, who were mothers, or family nearby. I started dropping by her house in the evening on my way home from the office. Gradually, the mother began to relax and feel more in control. When she went back to work, after finding a competent baby sitter, she was more like her old self and the baby was thriving.

- ✓ Join a new moms' group, the La Leche League, a Gymboree class, or a moms' fitness class.
- ✓ Join a singles' or parents' group.
- ✓ Get to know your neighbors.
- ✓ Find a church or other religious home and meet other parents.
- ✓ Take a class to meet new friends.
- ✓ Try one of the many parent chat rooms online to meet other mothers and ask questions.
- ✓ Find a new hobby or start a fun project.
- ✓ Get involved with some kind of community group if you are not working outside the house.
- ✓ Join a book group as a way to meet friends.
- ✓ Take walks with your baby to a park or community center. You'll probably meet other mothers there.
- ✓ Find a favorite coffee shop.
- ✓ Get to know the personnel in your neighborhood stores. They can be a great resource.
- ✓ Ask for help when you need it. A great deal of help is available but you have to be willing to ask for it.
- ✓ Find daily or weekly help. The pediatrician may have suggestions, as will other mothers. Be sure to check carefully on a baby sitter or childcare person's background and medical history.

SECTION 1: Babies and Infants (17)

CONSTIPATION

A three-day-old infant, I had not seen previously, was brought to my office. The parents were concerned the baby had not had a bowel movement since birth. The mother was nursing the infant, which seemed to be going well, but the baby fussed a great deal.

On looking at the baby, I was concerned about the lack of bowel movements and the infant's fussiness. When I examined the anus, it looked normal. However, when I inserted my smallest gloved finger, I felt a constricting band. With gentle pressure, the band released and considerable stool expelled. The baby had a congenital band inside the bowel. These are occasionally present and after the rectal examination, the infant had no further problem with constipation or fussiness. I was so glad the parents had consulted me when they did. Otherwise, major problems could have developed.

- ✓ Watch that bowel movements occur from day one.
- ✓ Try not to worry if soft stools occur only every few days. This may be normal.
- ✓ Watch and remember what you eat if you are nursing. A nursing baby may have several stools a day depending on the mother's diet.
- ✓ Keep track for a few days of your baby's pattern of bowel movements.
- ✓ Give diluted juice between feedings, as well as extra water, to help make the stools softer.
- ✓ Watch for severe constipation. This can be a sign of wheat intolerance or celiac disease.
- ✓ Be aware that applesauce and bananas are constipating; other fruits can make the stools softer.
- ✓ Note any bright red blood in a bowel movement. This can mean a crack or fissure by the anus.
- ✓ Watch for constipation with a poor weight gain and a listlessness. This can be a sign of low thyroid hormone (hypothyroidism). A blood test would be necessary to determine this.
- ✓ Be aware that constipation can be a problem in a floppy baby born with a muscle disease.

MEDICAL CONCERNS

A 5-month-old infant was brought into my office for the first time. The baby had not had regular medical care but had been delivered in a rural area by a midwife. The young parents had no support system and no prior experience with babies. They didn't realize the infant was quite delayed in development, had poor weight gain and seemed listless.

The baby's skin was rough and the parents said that he had hard, infrequent stools. After taking a history and doing an examination, I ordered a routine blood count, urinalysis, and test for thyroid function.

The test results were a surprise because they showed that the baby had hypothyroidism and needed thyroid replacement. Also, he was anemic and needed some iron supplement. Gradually, with medication, the baby made dramatic progress. If the parents had delayed seeing me much longer, developmental delay could have resulted.

- ✓ Note that poor weight gain or too rapid weight gain are both of concern.
- ✓ See a physician immediately if a baby is listless.
- ✓ Watch for any evidence of a poor suck.
- ✓ See a doctor is there are breathing problems.
- ✓ Consult a family doctor or pediatrician if there is a fever.
- ✓ See the baby's doctor immediately if there is little movement of the arms or legs.
- ✓ Visit a doctor's office immediately if there is prolonged jaundice or a yellow color of the skin and eyes.
- ✓ Have the baby's doctor investigate oozing or signs of infection around the navel.
- ✓ See the baby's doctor if there is pus oozing from the eyes.
- ✓ Try massage at the corner of the eye near the nose if there is an obstructed tear duct. Warm compresses may help also. **This way surgery may be avoided.**
- ✓ Make an immediate call to a physician if there is high-pitched or non-stop crying.
- ✓ Don't be afraid to call your doctor, even on a weekend if you are worried.
- ✓ Insist that you need to speak to your baby's doctor or the doctor on-call or ask that the physician call you back. "The squeaky wheel does get the grease."

SAFETY

A young mother called me frantically early on a Sunday morning saying her six-week-old baby had rolled from a low couch onto the floor. She said that the baby cried immediately but seemed to be okay. I asked her to meet me at the office, since we were both five minutes away.

On examination the baby seemed fine, so I decided to watch her for any problems. The fact that she had cried right away and had rolled from a low couch onto a thick carpet helped my decision. I would have kept her overnight in the hospital and obtained an X-ray of her head if she had dropped from a distance onto a hard surface. On follow-up during the day and for several years, there were no subsequent problems.

- ✓ Insist on X-rays if an infant is dropped or falls. Hospital observation may be necessary.
- ✓ Note signs of a head injury after a fall: loss of consciousness, poor color, and any evidence of bruising.
- ✓ Don't ever leave an infant alone on a changing table, bed or couch.
- ✓ Put an infant in an approved car seat for even a quick trip.
- ✓ Don't use cribs with cutouts in the foot or head of the bed.
- ✓ Use only flame resistant clothing.
- ✓ Have a smoke detector in a baby's room and check it twice a year.
- ✓ Place a functioning carbon monoxide detector in or near a baby's room.
- ✓ Be sure that your baby's mattress is firm and fits snugly in the crib.
- ✓ Don't have any dangling toys or cords that can ensnare a baby.
- ✓ Be sure pacifiers can't come apart.
- ✓ Don't use soft pillows or bedding in a baby's bed. These can be dangerous.
- ✓ Don't put ties or necklaces around a baby's neck.
- ✓ Check for small removable parts on toys.
- ✓ Use gates to block access to areas of danger.
- ✓ Watch for clothing with drawstrings that can catch on something and cause choking.
- ✓ Put babies to sleep on their backs not sides or abdomen.
- ✓ Know infant CPR.
- ✓ Check cribs at grandparents' homes, hotels, and motels to be sure they are safe.
- ✓ Be sure that the crib slats are no more than 2 and 3/8 inches apart.

DAYCARE

A professional mother placed her six-week-old infant in a nearby, licensed daycare center. She hadn't anticipated the frequent turnover in personnel or the lack of 1:1 attention. Ultimately, she and I both decided that the baby would get better care in an older woman's home. The woman was a retired nurse who had raised several children of her own and she was a wonderful find.

- ✓ Check and investigate thoroughly before choosing a daycare center.
- ✓ Be sure you get a good feeling about a daycare center.
- ✓ Check to be sure that a center has a good smell and is very clean.
- ✓ Ask if a daycare center is licensed.
- ✓ Inquire if the caretakers have emergency training, i.e. CPR.
- ✓ Ask what kind of training or background the caretakers have.
- ✓ Find out how close it is to the nearest emergency room, doctor or hospital.
- ✓ Ask about the ratio of babies or children to adults.
- ✓ Check on the policy about illness and if a sick child is sent home.
- ✓ Talk to parents of other infants and children in a daycare center prior to enrolling an infant or child.
- ✓ Drop in unexpectedly.
- ✓ Leave your contact numbers and those of a close friend, relative and the baby's doctor.
- ✓ Ask how long the daycare has been operating.
- ✓ Find out how many infants or children are cared for each day.
- ✓ Be sure the caretakers have had good background checks.

FINDING AND HIRING CHILDCARE WORKER

The neighbor of one of my new mothers called to say that she was worried about her friend's new baby in the flat below. The infant's mother had recently gone back to work after a leave of absence and had hired a new baby sitter. The kind neighbor had knocked on the door of the flat below and was concerned that the baby sitter seemed confused. Also the kitchen floor was littered with cereal.

The infant's mother couldn't be reached, so I hurried to the house to check the baby girl. The infant seemed fine and was in her bassinet. However, the baby sitter was groggy and confused. She said that she didn't feel well and would go to a friend's house if the nice neighbor upstairs would take the baby.

Later, I discovered the sitter had had a convulsion or seizure that morning and had a seizure disorder for which she refused medication. The new mother did check in a bit later and said she had asked the sitter about medical problems, but had not thought to get a letter from the woman's doctor. Fortunately, the infant wasn't hurt, but we all shuddered thinking about what the consequences could have been.

Finding a Sitter:
- ✓ Place an ad in the local newspaper listing specific needs such as: "Working mother desires motherly woman to care for infant **References required, light cooking, no housework**".
- ✓ Call a nanny or sitter employment service.
- ✓ Call senior centers for referrals.
- ✓ Network with other parents.
- ✓ Call church or other religious offices for referrals.
- ✓ Call a college employment service.
- ✓ Look at parenting newspapers.

Hiring a Sitter:
- ✓ Check on two or more references.
- ✓ Ask about medical problems and the date of the last chest X-ray or tuberculin skin test and request a new one if the test is more than a year old.
- ✓ Ask for a letter from the applicant's physician.
- ✓ Talk to one or two previous employers.

EATING

A new mother, who was bottle-feeding her baby, complained that the infant kept spitting up the milk. After I examined Jed, I watched the mother give him a bottle. The milk seemed to come out much too quickly, so we tried a nipple with a smaller hole. Both mother and baby were much happier and no further spitting up occurred.

___

- ✓ Watch that milk goes easily through a nipple and doesn't gush out.
- ✓ Be sure that a nipple hole isn't too small or too big. Some babies have a vigorous suck, whereas others, particularly premature babies, may have a weaker one.
- ✓ A pacifier can be used to space feedings.
- ✓ Note that spitting up can be caused by allergies.
- ✓ Put a baby in an upright position, as in an infant seat, for twenty minutes after a feeding to help prevent spitting up.
- ✓ Add one new food at a time.
- ✓ Offer single foods, not mixtures, when foods are first offered
- ✓ Give babies who are big eaters more than just milk.
- ✓ Add cereal to a baby's bottle to thicken feedings if a baby is a spitter.
- ✓ Watch for forceful vomiting. If this occurs after two or more feedings, it could indicate a problem.

EMERGENCIES

A 3-month-old baby was brought to my office with a fever of 103 degrees and a history of vomiting for two days. The parents had been traveling and hadn't checked the infant's temperature. Since the baby was nursing, the mother thought she had probably eaten something that was upsetting the infant. The parents didn't realize how very ill the baby was.

I immediately hospitalized the child, performed a spinal tap, as well as other tests, and started antibiotics. How glad I was that I had acted quickly when the lab results showed the baby had meningitis. Fortunately, the baby did well and had no residual problems.

A listless baby and/or a feverish small one should be seen immediately by a pediatrician or family doctor, <u>not</u> an ER doctor.

Other emergencies include:
- ✓ Loss of consciousness
- ✓ Convulsion or seizure
- ✓ Prolonged vomiting or diarrhea
- ✓ Severe, uncontrolled bleeding
- ✓ Inability to breathe
- ✓ Head injury with loss of consciousness
- ✓ Eye injury
- ✓ Fracture of a bone
- ✓ Choking
- ✓ Bright red blood
- ✓ Listlessness
- ✓ Excessive sleeping

NOTE: A rectal thermometer should be in any home where there is an infant. Rectal temperatures are easy to obtain and give accurate readings when done correctly. (Hold the baby's legs up and together with one hand while inserting the Vaseline-covered rectal thermometer into the anus with the other.) *If you are worried about your baby for any reason, <u>insist</u> on seeing a pediatrician or family doctor.*

INFORMATION FOR CHILDCARE WORKERS

A mother called one day saying there had been a sudden, unexpected family death and she was going to have to be gone for a few days. She said a sitter would be caring for the baby. She wanted me to know, in case there was a problem. I said I would check with the sitter and asked that the woman have all the information listed below. The mother was grateful for the list.

- ✓ Leave all your phone numbers for a sitter.
- ✓ Leave a list of telephone numbers of close friends, nearby grandparents, and your child's doctor.
- ✓ Leave close neighbors' names and telephones numbers.
- ✓ Post the telephone numbers of the doctor, dentist, police, fire department, and ambulance. Be sure it is in a place that can be easily seen.
- ✓ Leave a list of the baby's general routine.
- ✓ Make a list of the baby's food likes and dislikes and any allergies.
- ✓ List any medications taken; the dose, their location, and the time to be given.
- ✓ Note location of fire extinguishers.
- ✓ Note location and instructions for the furnace thermostat or wall heaters.
- ✓ Leave special instructions for the washer, dryer, dishwasher, and stove.
- ✓ Post the location of the first aid kit.
- ✓ Be sure the sitter can communicate if there is an emergency.
- ✓ Leave money for emergencies.
- ✓ *Have friends or neighbors drop by unexpectedly and be sure they have your cell phone or other out of town numbers.*

SECTION 1: Babies and Infants

FINDING A DOCTOR

A former parent called one day from Seattle asking if I could help to find a pediatrician for her new baby. She had had bad experiences with two previous ones because they wanted their office staff to answer all the questions and it was difficult to get an appointment to see the doctor. They also wanted her to see the nurse practitioner and she was not willing to do that. The mother asked me what questions she should ask to check out a new doctor. I did some research about doctors in her vicinity and had the following questions faxed to her.

- ✓ Ask if the doctor is part of a health plan and refers only to doctors in the HMO.
- ✓ Inquire how often the doctor is on-call at night and weekends and who covers when he or she is gone. Does another pediatrician see the children or are they seen by ancillary medical personnel? Also does the doctor just refer parents to an emergency room after hours or on weekends instead of seeing the baby himself or herself??
- ✓ Ask if in an emergency, if the doctor meets you in the ER or instead has the ER doctor see your child. (Emergency room doctors are fine for acute trauma, but not for most pediatric problems.)
- ✓ Find out who answers questions when you call; a nurse or can you speak to the doctor. Remember that you might not be told the truth about this and may have to learn the hard way.
- ✓ Ask if the doctor prescribes antibiotics over the phone or insists on seeing your baby. Kids must be examined before antibiotics are prescribed because a serious illness could be missed.
- ✓ Find out if the doctor has one or more offices and how many days a week he or she is in each one. A second office could be at a great distance.
- ✓ Ask about fees for routine and other visits and if the office staff will bill insurance companies.
- ✓ Check on the doctor's credentials. Is he or she a M.D. or D.O?
- ✓ Inquire if the doctor is board certified in his or her specialty. (This means specific tests have been passed after the training requirements are completed.)
- ✓ Find out how close the office is to a hospital and what hospital is used. In an emergency, it is important that a doctor can arrive quickly at the hospital.
- ✓ Check on the amount of time the doctor allots to each patient.
- ✓ Find out how close the doctor's office is to your house.
- ✓ Look to see that the office is clean and pleasant.
- ✓ Note if the office staff are pleasant and helpful.

CHOOSING AN HMO OR HEALTH INSURANCE

A newborn baby girl, Iris, was born with a dislocated hip. The infant's HMO doctor referred them to the orthopedist in their group who saw both children and adults. He was not a pediatric orthopedist or one with special training in children's disorders. The father called one day and was very upset saying they understood it was important to find an orthopedist with lots of experience in treating baby's hip problems. I agreed and gave them the names of two good pediatric orthopedists, who were not in their HMO. The parents were not able to get referrals to either of the doctors and decided to change health plans. The father called again saying he needed to know what questions he should ask before changing plans. The parents could have appealed the ruling about seeing an outside orthopedist but decided it was too important to get another orthopedist quickly.

- ✓ Ask the cost of premiums.
- ✓ Ask about any restrictions.
- ✓ Ask if there are co-payments and how much are they.
- ✓ Ask if out of state emergencies are paid for.
- ✓ Find out what surgeries are paid for
- ✓ Inquire if prescriptions are paid for or if there is a limit.
- ✓ Find out what hospitalizations are covered.
- ✓ Be sure each family member is covered.
- ✓ Ask if any conditions are excluded from coverage.
- ✓ Find out if there are restrictions about which specialists can be seen.
- ✓ Check if medical equipment is covered.
- ✓ Ask about the appeal process if coverage is denied.
- ✓ Find out how long an HMO has been in business.
- ✓ Inquire about who owns an HMO.
- ✓ Get a list of physicians included in the plan or under the insurance.

SECTION 1: Babies and Infants (27)

TWINS/MULTIPLE BIRTHS

A mother brought in her twin baby girls. Both were thriving but the mother seemed worried. When I asked how things were going, she said, "I'm concerned about my older little girl. She doesn't seem to like the babies and has actually pinched one of them. What can I do to help her?"

My answer was, "When twins or triplets are born and there is an older child, it is important a great deal of one-to-one attention is given that child. Remember that he or she has been the center of attention and suddenly the twins or triplets are the 'stars'. This is hard for any child to accept or understand. Special treats, extra time with each parent or grandparents and asking the child to help with the babies will all pay off. Older children love feeling big and responsible and like to help. Limits and appropriate discipline are still important even with lots of special attention."

- ✓ Always have lots of extra supplies. You'll need them!
- ✓ Treat each twin as a distinct personality.
- ✓ Avoid identical clothes, hairstyles, furniture, or color schemes.
- ✓ Be sure the twins have playmates. Twins often want to play just with each other.
- ✓ Many develop their own codes and language and live in their own special world.
- ✓ Place the twins in separate classrooms, if possible when they start preschool or school.
- ✓ Join a twin parents' group or find a twin chat-room online.
- ✓ Be sure older children get lots of time and attention.
- ✓ Plan a few minutes time each day just for you. Twins take extra time and energy.
- ✓ Look for each twin's special abilities as they grow up and encourage these.
- ✓ Don't allow one twin to dominate the other, if possible.
- ✓ Be sure the other twin gets equal attention if one has problems.

TOYS

Sam, an eighteen-year-old was packed ready to leave for his freshman year in college. On the top of his suitcases, in a position of importance, sat the youth's well-worn, enormous teddy bear. Sam had received the bear when he was a baby from a good friend of his parents. There was no way Teddy was going to be left at home!

_____

- ✓ Soft, cuddly dolls and stuffed animals are special.
- ✓ Check all toys for detachable, small parts.
- ✓ Music boxes near the crib are soothing.
- ✓ Colorful mobiles above the crib are fun.
- ✓ One-piece rattles are safe toys.
- ✓ Brightly colored, small toys are the best.
- ✓ Too many toys are confusing.
- ✓ The Consumer website can give you lists of toys that are re-called.

SKIN CARE

Julia, a 1-month-old baby, had frequent diaper rashes. Her mother tried many different lotions and powders, but nothing helped. I suggested she use nothing but mild soap and cornstarch as a powder. The rash quickly disappeared.

- ✓ Use as few lotions and powders as possible
- ✓ Cornstarch can help clear diaper rashes.
- ✓ A daily bath is important.
- ✓ Wash the diaper area well after bowel movements and with diaper changes.
- ✓ Nylon and wool clothing may cause rashes.
- ✓ Cotton clothes are best for sensitive babies.
- ✓ Leave the diaper area open to the air for a little while.
- ✓ Washing clothes with detergents may cause problems.

BATHING

A young mother was exhausted and overwhelmed after her baby's birth and became very anxious about bathing Steven because he was so wiggly. Her husband came to the rescue one night after coming home from work. He took charge and had no problem bathing his son. After that, the evening bath became a ritual. The father and Steven both enjoyed their special time together.

- ✓ **Never** leave a baby alone in a bath.
- ✓ Test the water before a baby's bath.
- ✓ A warm bath will soothe a baby.
- ✓ Never take a baby into a Jacuzzi.
- ✓ A towel in the bottom of a tub prevents slipping.
- ✓ Have music playing to make a bathing easier.
- ✓ Have everything needed within easy reach.
- ✓ Have a hot water regulator for old houses.
- ✓ Don't answer the telephone or door bell during bathtime.

SECTION 1: Babies and Infants   (31)

CLOTHING

Heather, a 6-month-old baby girl, was elegantly dressed in a 100-year-old family christening dress, slip, and little hat. She usually was a good baby, but when it became warm in the church, she started crying. Her grandmother motioned to the young parents to take off the hat and let some air circulate under the dress. Once Heather was cooler, she stopped crying.

- ✓ Check that sleepwear is flame retardant.
- ✓ Drawstrings around the neck are unsafe.
- ✓ Babies may be unhappy with layers of clothes.
- ✓ Hats are important for both cold and hot days.
- ✓ Babies outgrow clothing very quickly.
- ✓ Babies' clothes can be found in next-to-new shops.
- ✓ Babies may use several changes of clothes each day.
- ✓ Soft shoes or stockings should be used when a baby starts pulling up, unless there is a rug.

TEETHING

A 5-month-old baby began to fuss and cry intermittently. The parents thought the baby was teething. The baby's grandmother was visiting and suggested a rectal temperature be taken. It was 103 degrees. The parents immediately took the baby to their pediatrician and a bad ear infection was found.

- ✓ Chilled teething rings are comforting.
- ✓ Try rubbing the baby's gums with a clean finger.
- ✓ Teething biscuits are helpful.
- ✓ Teething usually doesn't cause fevers.
- ✓ Some babies have no teething problem; other babies get very fussy.
- ✓ Check a rectal temperature if a baby cries for a prolonged period.

BURPING

A mother of infant twins found that one twin burped easily, but the other one had difficulty. The mother quickly learned she had to give the difficult burper special drops the baby's pediatrician had prescribed. It was the only way the mother could get both babies fed and burped.

- ✓ Some babies are easy to burp, some are not.
- ✓ On the shoulder burping works for most.
- ✓ Sitting a baby up on your lap and rubbing the tummy works for others.
- ✓ Medication is available to help difficult burpers.
- ✓ Keep a baby upright for twenty minutes after feeding.
- ✓ An upset baby may just need to be burped.
- ✓ Putting a baby across your lap and patting the back can help a burp come up.

SECTION 1: Babies and Infants (33)

PETS

A very upset mother brought her six-weeks-old baby to the office because a friend's cat had clawed the baby's arm. A small scratch was visible. On calling the friend's veterinarian, I was told that the cat had been checked recently and was up-to-date on all shots.

- ✓ Safeguard an infant from all pets.
- ✓ A jealous pet can bite a baby.
- ✓ Be sure pets have all their shots.
- ✓ Pets can transmit diseases.
- ✓ Infants can be allergic to pets.
- ✓ Have regular care for your pet.
- ✓ Cover a sandbox when not in use.
- ✓ Wash babies' hands after they crawl.
- ✓ A hook high up on the door will keep animals from the infant.

CHILDPROOFING YOUR HOUSE

A grandmother was concerned that her daughter-in-law and son hadn't made their house child-proofed for 9-month-old Jenny. Both parents thought they had plenty of time plenty of time to safeguard the house before their daughter started walking. One night after putting Jenny to bed, they sat down in their living room to have coffee. Hearing a voice, they were startled to see Jenny coming down the hall. She had climbed out of her crib and wanted company!

- ✓ Safety locks or bolts should be on all outside doors.
- ✓ Gates should be at the top and bottom of stairs.
- ✓ A playpen is a MUST and does <u>not</u> restrict development.
- ✓ Covers should be on all electrical outlets.
- ✓ Cover sharp corners on all low furniture.
- ✓ Install window locks.
- ✓ Put covers on or over floor heater vents.
- ✓ Protect access to wall heaters with a guard.
- ✓ Have a safe, sturdy fireplace screen.
- ✓ Keep matches and lighters up high.
- ✓ Empty low kitchen cupboards, bathrooms, and bedside tables of medicine or poisonous substances.

INFANTS WITH SPECIAL NEEDS

A two-weeks-old infant, born with muscle weakness, was in the hospital intensive care nursery. The parents asked for a consultation, which I was glad to provide. In reviewing the baby's chart, I discovered the parents had not been referred to the state program for children with problems. The hospital bill was already high and was increasing daily. The parents' insurance did not cover the infant and they would have had to declare bankruptcy. With some urgent calls to CCS, the California state program, and some arm-twisting, CCS agreed to cover the baby's costs from birth.

- ✓ Each state has a program to cover children with disabilities.
- ✓ Immediate referral is needed for long hospital stays.
- ✓ Insist the physicians in-charge speak to you often.
- ✓ Take frequent breaks away from the hospital.
- ✓ Have a massage or other relaxing treat now and then.
- ✓ Eat enough protein and good food daily.
- ✓ Ask friends and family to help.
- ✓ Get to know each staff member by name.
- ✓ Get plenty of exercise.
- ✓ Beware of possible false information in medical journals and on the Internet.
- ✓ *Ask for a second opinion if the diagnosis is serious.*

INFANT SCHEDULES

A young mother came to the office. Fatigue lines were etched on her face and she looked ten years older than the last time I had seen her. "I can't keep up with Peter's feedings and schedule," she said. "He wants to nurse every 30 minutes. I'm exhausted."

- ✓ Full-term babies don't need to eat more often than every three to four hours.
- ✓ Feedings can be spaced with a pacifier or water.
- ✓ Rigid four-hour feedings don't work well for babies.
- ✓ Big babies usually are big eaters. Some need rice cereal in their bottles to fill them up.
- ✓ Babies should not be kept at the breast for more than 20 minutes or 10 minutes/side.
- ✓ Every baby needs to cry and fuss a little.

INFANT CPR

A young couple lost their first baby because of a genetic disorder. Before the second baby was due, I suggested they both should take a pediatric CPR course. They were much less anxious when the new baby arrived. Fortunately, the baby was fine.

- ✓ CPR courses are offered in some hospitals and by the Red Cross. See www.RedCross.org
- ✓ Websites offering CPR information are available.
- ✓ A monitor in the baby's room can decrease anxiety.
- ✓ It is dangerous for babies to ever sleep with parents.
- ✓ Babies should sleep on their backs to help prevent Sudden Infant Death or SIDS.
- ✓ Baby sitters or childcare workers should know CPR.
- ✓ If a baby stops breathing, be sure nothing is stuck in the throat.
- ✓ Avoid any food that can get lodged in the throat.

IMMUNIZATION TIPS

The parents of an autistic child refused to allow their younger children to have any immunizations. Both the mother and father were convinced that their son's autism had resulted from some of his baby shots. Unfortunately, the child had a severe case of measles that could have been prevented.

℞
_____

- ✓ Studies in prominent research centers have shown **Autism is not caused by immunizations.**
- ✓ Alert your baby's doctor to any fever or other reaction following an immunization.
- ✓ Check your baby's immunization record at each doctor's visit to be sure everything is up to date.
- ✓ Polio and other childhood diseases still occur in the U.S.
- ✓ Some doctors are lax about checking immunization dates.
- ✓ Know how to use and read a rectal thermometer.

GROWING STEPS

A mother was concerned that six-months-old, Nancy, was not sitting up. She was a fat, placid baby and on examination, I could find no muscle weakness or other problem. The grandmother assured the mother that the baby's daddy, a bright lawyer, had also been a fat, placid baby who was slow to sit and walk.

Rx

- ✓ Each baby will develop at his or her own pace.
- ✓ It is unwise to push a baby to sit or walk.
- ✓ Weak or floppy babies need to be checked by a pediatric neuromuscular specialist.
- ✓ Premature babies will be slow in development.
- ✓ Big babies may take longer to walk.
- ✓ **Hearing must be checked if a baby makes no sounds by three months.**
- ✓ Girl babies tend to develop speech before boys.
- ✓ If everything is done for a child, he or she may not try to do things for himself or herself.

HAVING FUN

"I didn't know having a baby would be this hard", a father said. "My wife and I never have fun any more. The baby has completely taken over our lives. Even if we could make time to go out, we'd be too tired. What can we do?"

Rx

- ✓ Put money aside for a weekly babysitter.
- ✓ Take mini-vacations.
- ✓ A night at a comedy club could help.
- ✓ Invite friends, who are fun, to come for a picnic, pot-luck, or glass of wine.
- ✓ Have a weekly date with your partner or spouse and don't talk about the baby.
- ✓ Call a senior center for babysitters.
- ✓ Hire a live-in college or graduate student.
- ✓ Trade babysitting with other parents.

SINGLE PARENTING

A military wife had a baby soon after she learned of her husband's death overseas. She had no close family nearby and knew she was in trouble. Money was also tight. The mother was new in the area and hadn't had time to make friends. She was also shy, so she felt very much alone.

Rx

- ✓ Find a single parent's support group.
- ✓ Find an online chat room.
- ✓ Let others help, but tell them what you need.
- ✓ Get exercise several times a week.
- ✓ Find a reliable babysitter.
- ✓ Don't try to be a super parent.
- ✓ Don't be afraid to ask for whatever help you need.
- ✓ Make new friends even though it may be hard to do.
- ✓ Go to a park where mothers congregate.
- ✓ Make friends at a gym.

MOTION

A small baby cried and cried. I couldn't find anything medically wrong and the parents didn't want to use medicine to quiet the baby. I made a house call to see if I could find answers. The baby was wide awake in a bassinet in a beautifully decorated room. Everything possible had been purchased for the baby, but one thing was missing, a rocking chair. Once the baby was rocked to sleep there were no more problems. I told the happy parents that mothers long ago knew motion was needed for some babies. Antique cradles were made to rock, so a baby could be lulled to sleep.

Rx

- A rocking chair in a baby's room is important.
- A car ride usually calms an upset baby.
- Approved baby swings can be life-saving.
- Walking with a baby can help parents and the baby.
- A rocking cradle can save the day.
- Too much motion can be as bad as too little.
- Gentle rocking in a quiet, dark room is the best.

SECTION 1: Babies and Infants

EQUIPMENT

A young couple were so excited about becoming parents that they immediately decorated a spare room. One set of grandparents provided a crib and the other a stroller. The parents also bought a new car. When an ultrasound revealed twins were on their way, the couple were excited, but dismayed. They realized their car was not big enough for a double stroller and other needed equipment. Also, they knew another crib, a different stroller, and two of everything would be needed. They weren't sure their house was big enough for so much equipment.

Rx

- ✓ Shop wisely and limit your purchases.
- ✓ Be sure any second-hand equipment is clean and safe.
- ✓ Check the Internet and catalogs for good buys.
- ✓ Be sure a crib's side rails are no more than 2 and 3/8 inches apart.
- ✓ Sturdy gates are needed at the top and bottom of stairs.
- ✓ A playpen is a MUST for safety reasons.
- ✓ A firm mattress in a crib is important.
- ✓ Many older parents have equipment to give or sell.

SOUND

A young mother brought her beautiful, first baby in to the office. The baby was unusually good and the mother said that no matter what noise was in the house, the baby didn't seem to mind. This concerned me, because most babies will react to loud noises. Some are disturbed by even minimal noises. I asked that the baby have her hearing tested in a pediatric hearing center. It was an important test because the baby was found to have congenital deafness.

Rx

- ✓ If a baby is not reacting to noise or sounds, a hearing test is needed, even if it was done after birth.
- ✓ Some babies need almost total quiet.
- ✓ Other babies sleep through anything.
- ✓ Sounds that are soothing to babies are
    - "White noise"
    - Music boxes
    - Bird sounds
    - Ocean waves
    - Water falls
    - Running streams
- ✓ Loud talking, TVs, and radios can be disturbing.

SECTION 1: Babies and Infants (43)

COLIC

When a little baby has the colic, it can be a frightening experience for parents or babysitters. As a young medical student, I was babysitting a couple's small baby. They didn't tell me she had colic, but I found out the hard way. I will never forget that night!

Rx

- ✓ Some colicky babies are allergic to milk.
- ✓ Nursing mothers should stop milk products to see if that helps.
- ✓ A pacifier may help.
- ✓ Gastric reflux is the cause in some babies.
- ✓ Elevating the head of the bed helps prevent reflux.
- ✓ Keep babies upright for twenty minutes after a feed.
- ✓ Motion and keeping a baby warm may help.
- ✓ Drugs, caffeine, herb teas and some foods bother nursing babies.
- ✓ Be sure there is no medical cause for the crying.

SUPPLIES

I was standing in line in a grocery store behind a thin, pale mother and small baby. The woman had a grocery cart filled with every possible kind of baby powder, soap, and lotion. For payment, she pulled out food stamps. I wanted so much to tell her that it wasn't necessary to use her food stamps for baby products. The fewer things used on a baby's skin, the better. I wished the mother had used her food stamps to buy some good food for herself.

Rx

- ✓ Check with older parents about needed supplies.
- ✓ Have lots of diapers, little shirts, and nightgowns.
- ✓ Baby bibs help keep clothes clean.
- ✓ A diaper bag is important to have.
- ✓ Check the Internet for good bargains.
- ✓ Expensive clothes will be quickly outgrown.
- ✓ Baby nail scissors are important.
- ✓ Diaper wipes are helpful.
- ✓ Don't buy unnecessary baby products.

PREMATURE BABIES

Mary was born three months early and was a tiny preemie. Her mother had stopped her marketing job just before the baby's birth. Daily she made the long trip to the hospital to sit by Mary's bed. When I made hospital rounds one morning, I found Mary almost falling asleep in her chair.

Rx

- ✓ Visiting a preemie is important, but long visits can be tiring and unhealthy for parents.
- ✓ A daily walk away from the hospital can help.
- ✓ Insist the doctors keep you up-to-date.
- ✓ Parents of preemies need to pamper themselves
- ✓ Let friends and family take your place and run errands.
- ✓ Have a weekly date with your mate.
- ✓ Husbands can feel left out when a preemie is born.
- ✓ Don't skimp on good meals.

SCHEDULES FOR WELL CHECKUPS

A couple brought in 4-month-old Cynthia. She had been born at home in the mountains and was never examined by a physician. The parents said they had had bad experiences with doctors. They were reluctant to bring the baby to see me, but she had come down with a bad cold and cough. I gave them antibiotics for Cynthia's bad cough and ear infection and talked to them about the importance of check-ups.

Rx

- ✓ Regular well-baby visits are important
- ✓ Doctors differ on the frequency of visits.
- ✓ Babies should be checked for hip dislocations and other congenital problems.
- ✓ Problems detected early have a better cure rate.
- ✓ Immunizations are extremely important.
- ✓ Well visits are important to discuss feedings, check weight gain, and signs of anemia.
- ✓ Even newborns can develop infections.
- ✓ Umbilical healing is important to check.
- ✓ Head size should be checked on each visit.

SECTION 1: Babies and Infants (47)

HOSPITALIZATIONS

A baby was being changed on a bed when the phone rang. The mother thought she had surrounded Norma with pillows to keep her from moving, but somehow the baby had managed to roll onto the wood floor. The terrified mother called me at once and I met her in the emergency room. The baby looked all right, though she was a little pale. A skull X-ray revealed a small fracture, so I admitted Norma for observation.

Rx

- ✓ It is better to be safe than sorry.
- ✓ Check your insurance or HMO policies regarding coverage for hospitalizations.
- ✓ Always check your hospital bill carefully.
- ✓ Elective surgeries may be denied and an appeal necessary.
- ✓ Insist that your baby's doctor speak with you daily.
- ✓ Don't be intimidated by insurance company personnel.
- ✓ Get to know the nursing and other staff by name.
- ✓ Someone should always be with a hospitalized child.

Section 2

TODDLER BEHAVIOR PROBLEMS

INCLUDES PARENTING PRESCRIPTIONS FOR:

FRUSTRATION AND COMMUNICATION DIFFICULTY 49

EATING PROBLEM AND CELIAC DISEASE..50

HYPERACTIVITY AND ADHD............51

WHINING AND CONGENITAL HEART DISEASE.................................52

UNUSUAL BEHAVIOR AND MILK ANEMIA...53

CRYING AND FOREIGN BODY.........54

IRRITABILITY AND DIABETES...........55

ACTING OUT AND PINWORMS.......56

UNHAPPY/HEARING PROBLEM.......57

ATTENTION GETTING AND FAMILY ILLNESS 58

SLEEP PROBLEMS/LONELINESS 58

BORED AND BRIGHT.........................59

IRRITABLE AND ALLERGIES 59

TEMPER TANTRUMS AND MARITAL PROBLEMS...........................60

CRYING AND FOREIGN BODY.........60

GROUCHY AND FAST FOOD DIET ...61

WITHDRAWING AND AUTISM 62

DIFFICULT AND SIBLING WITH A DISABILITY..63

UNHAPPY AND LACK OF SLEEP 64

ATTENTION SEEKING AND SPOILED 65

UPSET AND METABOLIC DISORDER..66

BREATH HOLDING AND OBESITY ...67

HEAD BANGING AND EMOTIONAL PROBLEMS...................68

UNHAPPY AND ABNORMAL KIDNEY..69

WHINING AND CONSTIPATION.....70

ANGER AND LACK OF ATTENTION...................................71

MOODY AND HUNGER.....................72

OUT OF CONTROL AND MEDICATION REACTION 73

HEAD BANGING AND VISION PROBLEM...74

MISBEHAVING AND BUSY/STRESSED PARENTS 74

TWITCHING AND LEARNING DISABILITY..75

FRUSTRATION AND HIGH EXPECTATIONS 76

NEUROTIC AND NEEDING AFFECTION...77

MISERABLE AND EAR INFECTIONS................................78

KICKING AND PARENTS DIVORCE 79

HITTING AND PARENTAL GRIEVING 80

HIGH STRUNG AND OVERSTIMULATION 81

WHY CHILDREN GET UPSET AND IRRITABLE..................................82

CHECKUP LIST TO HELP PREVENT IRRITABLE TODDLERS....83

FRUSTRATION AND COMMUNICATION DIFFICULTY

When the parents of 3-year-old boy, Larry, were asked to come for a conference at his preschool, they were upset and greatly concerned by what the principal told them. She said Larry was acting out so much they could no longer keep him at the school. She suggested the parents take him to see an educational psychologist and the psychologist found Larry had a severe communication problem. Apparently, he was so frustrated at not being able to communicate that he acted out. A speech assessment and therapy were advised.

Rx

- ✓ A child with a communication problem needs a hearing test in a pediatric hearing center.
- ✓ Assessment by a speech pathologist is needed for a child with communication problems.
- ✓ There are multiple reasons why a child acts out.
- ✓ An assessment by an educational psychologist is important for kids who act out.
- ✓ A pediatrician should be consulted to rule out medical problems.

EATING PROBLEM AND CELIAC DISEASE

It was an effort to get Connie, a two-year-old, up every morning, her parents said. She was irritable, didn't like to eat, wasn't growing well, or gaining weight. Connie's parents were beside themselves about what to do. On examination, she had a prominent tummy and looked sick and pale. I ordered several tests and the results were surprising. Connie had Celiac disease and was unable to tolerate wheat. Once all wheat products were removed from her diet, she began to act like a normal child, grow, and gain weight. She was no longer irritable.

Rx

- ✓ Celiac disease can be associated with either loose bowel movements or constipation.
- ✓ Multiple tests should be done if a child is irritable and not gaining weight.
- ✓ Wheat is present in many foods. Labels should be read carefully.
- ✓ Get a second opinion if one doctor can't find the answers for a child who seems ill.
- ✓ Cookbooks and resources are available for Celiac patients.

SECTION 2: Toddler Behavior Problems (51)

HYPERACTIVITY AND ADHD

No matter what the parents tried, Kevin was always in trouble. He was in trouble at his preschool and at home was constantly on the go and into everything. His parents brought him to see me because they were at the end of their patience. Kevin seemed unusually bright, but had trouble sitting still. I suspected that he was a child with an attention-deficit syndrome or ADHD. On testing by an excellent child psychologist, this proved to be the case and he responded beautifully to small doses of medication.

Rx

- ✓ Hyperactivity in a child can have several causes.
- ✓ Blood tests should be done for several disorders.
- ✓ An educational psychologist may need to do special testing.
- ✓ Bright children may just be bored.
- ✓ Hyperactivity can be just attention getting.
- ✓ More structure and discipline may be needed.
- ✓ Anxiety may accompany ADHD.
- ✓ Children with developmental delay are often hyperactive.

WHINING AND CONGENITAL HEART DISEASE

A mother brought her two-year-old son, George, to see me. They had recently moved from Las Vegas. The parents knew George had Down's Syndrome, but didn't understand why other children with the same syndrome seemed happy while George whined and was irritable. When I examined the child, a heart murmur was audible. I knew congenital heart disease was often present in Down's children and a pediatric heart doctor confirmed that George had a heart problem. After heart surgery, George was a different child.

Rx

- ✓ A child with a genetic syndrome should be checked for associated problems..
- ✓ If one congenital problem is present in a child, other physical problems may be found.
- ✓ An agency associated with a particular syndrome may offer help, support and literature.
- ✓ A pediatrician or geneticist familiar with a particular syndrome should always be consulted.

SECTION 2: Toddler Behavior Problems

UNUSUAL BEHAVIOR AND MILK ANEMIA

A mother brought two-year-old Jessica in with the complaint of behavior problems. When I took a detailed history, I discovered that Jessica's diet was almost entirely milk. She filled up on milk and didn't like regular food. A blood count revealed an iron deficiency anemia. This happens often in two-year-olds who become addicted to milk. When a child fills up on milk, there may not be an appetite for solid foods. They also may be very constipated which can decrease the appetite.

Rx

- ✓ A complete blood count (CBC) should always be done in a child with behavior problems.
- ✓ A two-year-old needs no more than sixteen ounces of milk.
- ✓ No two-year-old needs milk at night.
- ✓ Never leave a bottle of milk in a child's crib.
- ✓ Milk should be offered only with meals.
- ✓ Juice and water can be given between meals.
- ✓ Two-year-olds are particularly prone to milk anemia.
- ✓ If constipation is present, the child's doctor should be consulted.

CRYING AND FOREIGN BODY

Rachel and her mother lived with the grandmother. She had always been a good child until the last two or three weeks, the mother said. For some reason, Rachel had started crying and whining, but couldn't tell her mother if anything hurt. On examining the child, I noticed she seemed to favor her left leg. .Otherwise, I could not find a problem. I ordered an X-ray of the leg and foot and everyone was amazed to see a small needle in the child's foot. I found out that the grandmother sewed almost daily and Rachel spent a lot of time with her.

Rx
_____

- ✓ Small children have difficulty localizing pain.
- ✓ If a child limps there is usually a medical reason.
- ✓ Often the cause of pain is in the joint above where the pain seems to be.
- ✓ An X-ray can often provide a diagnosis.
- ✓ MRIs are often requested when an X-ray would do.
- ✓ Rheumatoid arthritis (JRA) can cause a child to limp.
- ✓ X-rays of the hip are important with limping in a child.
- ✓ Blood tests for JRA may be negative early in the disease.
- ✓ A slit-lamp examination of the eyes should be done in any limping child to help rule out JRA.

SECTION 2: Toddler Behavior Problems (55)

IRRITABILITY AND DIABETES

A grandmother was concerned that her grandson seemed more and more unhappy and irritable. She also noticed a smell in her bathroom and stickiness on the floor around the toilet. After examining Norman, I quickly checked a urine specimen. There was a strong positive reaction for sugar, so I ordered an immediate or stat blood sugar. This was markedly elevated. Norman was hospitalized and once the insulin dose was regulated, Norman became a happy child despite his diabetes.

Rx

- ✓ Childhood or early onset diabetes can cause irritability.
- ✓ A urinalysis is a simple, inexpensive test.
- ✓ Every child should have a <u>yearly</u> urinalysis.
- ✓ A family history of diabetes is important to note.
- ✓ Diabetes has three principal symptoms: increased thirst, hunger, and urination.
- ✓ Weight loss can also accompany diabetes.

ACTING OUT AND PINWORMS

I saw Freddy for a preschool examination. His mother said she had been taking him to a child psychiatrist because he was always rubbing against objects and acting out. On examination, Freddy's skin around the anus appeared red and irritated. I asked the mother to check for pinworms that night and she called at ten p.m. very upset. Her report was that pinworms were swarming around Freddy's anus. His irritability and acting out stopped after he was given pinworm medicine.

Rx

- ✓ Pinworms are common in little children.
- ✓ The pinworms come out of the anus at night and can be seen using a flashlight.
- ✓ Children need to wash their hands after playing in a sandbox or at a park.
- ✓ Other family members are often affected.
- ✓ Bed linen should be washed often.
- ✓ Pinworms can be a cause of stomach pain.
- ✓ A stool specimen should be checked for parasites.

UNHAPPY AND HEARING PROBLEM

This three-year-old child was picked on other children and always seemed whining and unhappy. The parents had had multiple tests done and thought she was developmentally delayed. On examination, I found both ear canals occluded with copious amounts of impacted wax (cerumen). The mother said she cleaned the child's ears with Q-tips. It took a great deal of time to remove the large amounts of wax from Sylvia's ear canals, but a different child got up from the examining table. Suddenly, Sylvia could hear. She was not delayed, but had had trouble hearing and reacted by acting out.

Rx

- ✓ Using Q-tips in children's ear canals is unwise.
- ✓ Every irritable, unhappy child should have their ears examined carefully and a hearing test.
- ✓ Every child thought to be delayed should have a hearing test.
- ✓ Any child with a speech problem should have a hearing test.
- ✓ Be sure your pediatrician or family doctor is seeing the ear drums. It takes time to clean wax out of the ears.
- ✓ Children stick things in their ear canals like beads.
- ✓ Insects sometimes get into a child's ear canal.

ATTENTION GETTING AND FAMILY ILLNESS

Ben's mother became bed-ridden with multiple sclerosis. The father found it difficult to keep housekeepers and Ben's mother could do little parenting. The father worked long hours, so Ben started acting out. He was fine at preschool, but at home did everything he could to get attention. The problem was finally solved by having a live-in graduate student who spent time with Ben.

Rx

- ✓ It is hard for little children to understand a parent's illness or disability.
- ✓ Relatives, friends, and neighbors will often be pleased to help out, if asked.
- ✓ No parent should be hesitant to ask for help.
- ✓ Senior centers, church or synagogue personnel may know people who can help.
- ✓ A bedridden parent should be involved as much as possible with his or her children.
- ✓ Some good books are available for kids with ill or disabled parents.

SLEEP PROBLEMS AND LONELINESS

Marjorie was a beautiful little two and one-half year old. Her father worked during the day and her mother worked at night in a hospital. The little girl had no playmates and needed to be quiet during the day, so her mother could sleep. Before long, the child started acting out, not sleeping well, and generally misbehaving. No playmates were close by and the parents couldn't afford a preschool. A grandparent came to the rescue and paid for Marjorie to go to a neighbor's house for several hours daily.

Rx

- ✓ No little child should be expected to be completely quiet during the day.
- ✓ Many nursery and preschools have scholarships or sliding fee scales.
- ✓ Check parent newsletters for good childcare.
- ✓ Other parents may have suggestions.
- ✓ A live-in college student could be a resource.
- ✓ Little children need attention and playmates.

SECTION 2: Toddler Behavior Problems

BORED AND BRIGHT

This four-year old couldn't wait to start school. He did well initially in his preschool, but then the parents began to get complaints that he was misbehaving. I suggested he see an excellent child psychologist. She did some testing and found Mark was unusually bright and could read. When the teacher let the boy read and do some special projects, there was no more acting out.

Rx

- ✓ Extremely bright children need to be kept busy with books, art, music, or projects.
- ✓ A visit to a good child psychologist may be worth its weight in gold.
- ✓ Not all child psychologists know how to do the appropriate tests for kids.
- ✓ Computer time should be limited for little children, as should all electronic devices.
- ✓ Every child needs some daily exercise.

IRRITABLE AND ALLERGIES

Megan was an unhappy, irritable toddler. There was a strong family history of allergy, so I suspected her frequent colds and irritability could be due to allergy. An excellent pediatric allergist found that Megan was sensitive to many things. Once allergy precautions were taken and some foods eliminated, the little girl became a very different and happy child.

Rx

- ✓ Allergic children frequently dislike milk.
- ✓ Dark circles under the eyes and rubbing the nose are often signs of allergy.
- ✓ A pediatric allergist should always be consulted, if a child may be allergic.
- ✓ Frequent colds often occur with allergy.
- ✓ Allergic children may be very irritable.
- ✓ Frequent ear infections may be due to allergy.

TEMPER TANTRUMS AND MARITAL PROBLEMS

A mother and father came to see me saying they were having marital problems, which seemed to be affecting their daughter, Kelsey. She was having temper tantrums, clinging to her mother and having separation anxiety. I suggested some counseling for the parents. They did get counseling, but the marriage ended in divorce. With some good parenting at both houses, Kelsey stopped acting out and no longer had separation anxiety.

Rx

- ✓ Children are very sensitive to parental tension.
- ✓ Two happy houses are better than one angry one.
- ✓ Family counseling may help in tense situations.
- ✓ Children often do well with a play therapist.
- ✓ Firm rules are needed at each house.
- ✓ Parents should not try to buy kids with gifts.
- ✓ Parents need to put their kids' welfare above all else.
- ✓ Communication between parents is important.

CRYING AND FOREIGN BODY

Peggy cried frequently, had intermittent fevers, and seemed miserable. On examination, I noticed pus coming from her vagina. An X-ray revealed a small safety pin was lodged there. The mother admitted the little girl often stuck things in her ears, nose, and also it seemed her vagina. Once the pin was removed Peggy had no more fevers or crying.

Rx

- ✓ Little children often poke small objects in every orifice.
- ✓ Pus coming from the nose, ears, rectum, or vagina should always be investigated.
- ✓ Intermittent fevers in kids must be investigated.
- ✓ Chest and neck X-rays should always be done for a persistent cough. A foreign body may be present that a child has swallowed.

GROUCHY AND FAST FOOD DIET

A little boy was seen who was irritable, whined frequently, and complained of muscle aches. His family doctor thought he had a muscle disease. In taking a history, I discovered the family lived almost entirely on fast foods. The mother worked long hours and was a single parent. No vitamins were taken and few fruits or vegetables were eaten. Once the mother changed the family's eating habits, Spencer became a happy child with no more muscle aches. His muscle disease was cured!

Rx

- ✓ The saying is true that we are what we eat.
- ✓ All children need a daily multi-vitamin.
- ✓ Protein, fruits, and vegetables should be given daily.
- ✓ Fast foods contain much fat and carbohydrate.
- ✓ A good breakfast is important for kids.
- ✓ Children can help shop and plan healthy meals.
- ✓ Shopping for the week can be done on a weekend.
- ✓ Preparing meal plans on weekends is helpful.
- ✓ Water or juice should replace soft drinks.

WITHDRAWING AND AUTISM

Adrian was a handsome two-year-old. His parents couldn't have been more delighted when he was born. Their joy turned to worry when the little boy began more and more to live in a world of his own. He was often angry, didn't want to be touched, and had frequent repetitive motions. The family doctor said Adrian was just a normal two-year-old. The parents knew something was wrong and sought a second opinion. After extensive testing, the specialist told the parents that Adrian was autistic. They were heartbroken.

Rx

- ✓ Get a second opinion if you are worried about a child.
- ✓ Parents are the experts with their children.
- ✓ Always trust your gut feelings.
- ✓ Sometimes even a third opinion is necessary.
- ✓ Autism is characterized by poor interaction with others, poor eye contact, and often repetitive motions.
- ✓ Autism is not caused by immunizations.
- ✓ Asperger's syndrome is a milder form of autism.
- ✓ Autism is now placed in so-called autism spectrum disorders category or ASD.

DIFFICULT AND SIBLING WITH A DISABILITY

Three-year-old Bridget was becoming increasingly difficult her parents said. She was acting out, having temper tantrums and breath-holding spells. An older brother used a wheelchair because of muscular dystrophy. The parents said they just couldn't handle any more problems. I suspected Bridget was trying to get her parents' attention, which proved to be the case. Once each parent spent some one-to-one time with the little girl, the problems ceased.

Rx

- ✓ Children who have a sibling with a disability are either very good or act out to get attention.
- ✓ Siblings of a child with a disability often have guilt that they are normal or caused the disability.
- ✓ Spending one to one time and really communicating with the siblings is extremely important.
- ✓ A newsletter for siblings of disabled kids is available at: The Sibling Information Network -203-344-7500

UNHAPPY AND LACK OF SLEEP

Henry was a nervous, tired, unhappy looking child. When I asked about the details of the family's life I discovered the reason. Both parents worked long hours, so the babysitter let Henry stay up to see his parents. He was so tired by then he had trouble falling asleep. The parents said they couldn't afford to give up their jobs and didn't know what to do. The solution we worked out was hard, but seemed the only one possible. Henry started spending the week with his grandparents and saw his parents on the weekend. Eventually, the parents were able to work shorter hours.

Rx

- ✓ Little children need a regular, early bedtime.
- ✓ Some children require more sleep than others.
- ✓ Tired children and tired parents equal trouble.
- ✓ Children get sick more easily, if they are tired.
- ✓ Kids who are tired do poorly in school.
- ✓ Tired children have more accidents.
- ✓ Kids who are tired get irritable and angry.
- ✓ Tired children don't eat well.

SECTION 2: Toddler Behavior Problems (65)

ATTENTION SEEKING AND SPOILED

Sharon was a beautiful toddler with over-indulgent parents and grandparents. No matter what she wanted, it was immediately purchased. Her room was full of toys, beautiful clothes, and books. When she started preschool, Sharon expected the teacher to do her bidding, as did her family. It was a rude shock when she realized this wasn't going to happen. Then Sharon began acting out at school to get attention. Finally, the principal asked the parents to keep her at home. She was too disruptive in the classroom.

Rx

- ✓ Spoiling a child leads to problems for everyone.
- ✓ Spoiling a little child will create problems as a teen.
- ✓ Discipline is love. Spoiling is _not_ love.
- ✓ It is easier to spoil kids than to parent them.
- ✓ All children need to have some wishes unfilled.
- ✓ A child who is given everything will become bored.
- ✓ Earning treats makes them more valuable.
- ✓ Every child needs to have something to wish for.
- ✓ Chores give a child a feeling of importance.

UPSET AND METABOLIC DISORDER

Mary was a small, unusual looking child. She had breath-holding spells, whined a lot, and got upset. In addition, the parents noticed a strong odor to her body and feet. There was little to see on examination but the unusual body odor was very evident. The mother had had a series of miscarriages and Mary was the parents first, much anticipated child. I referred the child to a pediatric metabolic specialist and after a series of tests in the hospital, an unusual metabolic disorder was diagnosed.

Rx

- ✓ Metabolic disorders are abnormalities in the way chemical changes take place in the body.
- ✓ There are very few pediatric metabolic experts in the United States.
- ✓ Complex testing is needed to establish the diagnosis of a metabolic disorder.
- ✓ An unusual body odor is a tip-off to a metabolic disorder.
- ✓ More and more metabolic disorders can now be diagnosed.
- ✓ Many screening tests are now done on newborns for these disorders.
- ✓ A second or even third opinion may be needed.
- ✓ Some metabolic disorders are treatable.

SECTION 2: Toddler Behavior Problems

BREATH HOLDING AND OBESITY

Mildred was a large baby at birth and each year seemed to get bigger and bigger. Her parents didn't think they were overfeeding her, but at her preschool, the child would have breath-holding spells if she didn't get to snack all morning. Her older sister told me that Mildred loved butter and since the parents owned a restaurant, the child would get one cook to butter her bread, lick it off, and then get another cook or helper to re-butter it. It was a large restaurant, so each one didn't know what the other one was doing. Once the parents laid down the law, the child lost weight and stopped having tantrums.

Rx

- ✓ Obese kids are often headed for unhappy futures.
- ✓ Obese kids are at risk for heart disease and diabetes.
- ✓ Fat kids are teased mercilessly.
- ✓ Overweight children usually have poor self-images.
- ✓ Overfeeding a child is not an act of love.
- ✓ Family eating habits may need to be changed.
- ✓ Grandparents or relatives may also be overfeeding a child.
- ✓ Keep a three-day record of everything a child eats.
- ✓ Cutting out fast foods can make a difference.
- ✓ Hospital dietitians can do consultations.

HEAD BANGING AND EMOTIONAL PROBLEMS

From birth, Alfred was an unhappy baby. As a toddler, he was a head banger, had breath-holding spells, set fires, and would hurt other children and small animals. A good child psychiatrist worked with the family and Alfred for awhile, but when the boy started destroying everything around him, the psychiatrist had him admitted to a home for emotionally disturbed children. There the boy received excellent psychiatric care.

Rx

- ✓ Some kids are born with emotional or psychiatric disorders.
- ✓ Children can have emotional disorders despite good parenting.
- ✓ An emotionally disturbed child may need institutional care.
- ✓ Good child psychiatrists are worth their weight in gold.
- ✓ It is best for kids with severe psychiatric disorders to be placed where they can have on-going professional care.
- ✓ Parents of disturbed kids need on-going support.
- ✓ If parents deny there is a problem with a child serious problems could develop.
- ✓ The siblings of a child with a psychiatric disorder need support.

SECTION 2: Toddler Behavior Problems (69)

UNHAPPY AND ABNORMAL KIDNEY

Juanita from birth was frequently ill, never seemed happy, and was difficult toddler. A series of blood and other tests did not reveal any problems. The parents were unwilling at first to have any other tests done. Finally, they allowed some kidney studies. These showed a greatly enlarged, abnormal kidney. Once the kidney was removed, the little girl became a much happier child.

Rx

- ✓ Congenital problems occur most frequently in the urinary tract (kidneys, bladder, ureters).
- ✓ Every child should have a yearly urinalysis.
- ✓ Little girls should have urinary studies after two urinary infections in the bladder or kidneys.
- ✓ Little boys should have a urinary-work-up after their first urinary infection by a pediatric urologist.
- ✓ Most children only urinate three to four times a day.
- ✓ Urinary frequency can be a sign of trouble
- ✓ Bed wetting can be a sign of urinary problems.

WHINING AND CONSTIPATION

Bettina was seen because of muscle weakness. She was an unhappy, whining child and her parents thought this was because she had a hard time keeping up with other children. When I examined her abdomen, I felt big lumps of stool. On rectal examination, I was puzzled how the child could go to the bathroom at all, since the stool was so hard. Once the constipation was under control, Bettina was a happy little girl despite her muscle disorder.

Rx

- ✓ A constipated child is usually an unhappy child.
- ✓ A child with muscle weakness is often constipated.
- ✓ Apples and bananas are constipating
- ✓ Juices and water help relieve constipation.
- ✓ Large amounts of milk are constipating.
- ✓ Cheese can be constipating.
- ✓ Most fruits, vegetables, and lettuce help bowel movements.
- ✓ Bran sprinkled on cereal or in muffins helps.
- ✓ A stool softener may need to be given.

ANGER AND LACK OF ATTENTION

A cute toddler was playing quietly in a dentist's waiting room. His mother was engrossed in a fashion magazine. After a while, the little boy picked up a children's book and asked his mother to read it to him. "In a while," the mother said. Again and again the little boy tried to get his mother's attention. Finally, he started throwing toys from the dentist's toy basket. Then he got his mother's attention!

Rx

- ✓ No child can be good all of the time.
- ✓ If kids are ignored, they will find ways to get attention.
- ✓ Use times alone with kids to read or talk to them.
- ✓ Children need to know they are important.
- ✓ Little children can play quietly for just so long.
- ✓ Some crayons and paper can help, if a parent is busy.
- ✓ Spending one-to one time with a child pays off greatly.
- ✓ Take along a favorite toy, book, or game for times when a child will need to be quiet.

MOODY AND HUNGER

James' mother found it hard to get up in the morning, she told me. Because of this, her little boy frequently went to school without any breakfast. Periodically, his preschool teachers reported James was moody or was difficult. Once the mother started giving James a breakfast peanut butter sandwich, she would make the night before, his disruptive behavior stopped.

Rx

- ✓ Hungry kids will be unhappy, irritable kids.
- ✓ Insist that your kids eat breakfast.
- ✓ Breakfast can be made the night before.
- ✓ Kids don't learn well when they are hungry.
- ✓ Kids get irritable without regular meals.
- ✓ Avoid foods with high sugar content.
- ✓ Don't depend on the school to feed your kids.
- ✓ Cheese, bananas, and peanut butter are good starters.

SECTION 2: Toddler Behavior Problems (73)

OUT OF CONTROL AND MEDICATION REACTION

A mother was going to fly across country to see an ill parent. Her doctor husband gave her some Phenobarbital tablets to give their toddler prior to take-off. Once the plane was in the air, the child was up and down, yelling, trying to get out of her seat. She was completely out of control. It was a terrible flight and the mother vowed never again to give Madeline medicine prior to a flight.

Rx

- ✓ Little children may become hyperactive with sedatives.
- ✓ Stimulants may have a sedating effect on little kids.
- ✓ Never give a child a new Rx away from home or on a plane.
- ✓ Medicine doses can vary even with the same size child.
- ✓ Parents should always check about possible Rx side effects.
- ✓ Adult medicines may not be OK for kids.
- ✓ Call a pharmacist if you have questions about medicines.
- ✓ Herbal medicines should not be given to children.

HEAD BANGING AND VISION PROBLEM

Ned was a head banger and always seemed unhappy. When I examined him, he seemed to be squinting. I asked his mother if he held books close to his face or sat close to the TV, "Yes", she said, "but I thought it was just a habit." The child had trouble seeing the office eye chart, so I referred him to a pediatric eye doctor. The specialist confirmed that Ned needed glasses. Once the boy became accustomed to the glasses, his disruptive behavior ceased.

Rx

- Headaches and eye strain can be manifested by squinting and irritability.
- Little children can't localize or vocalize pain.
- A yearly exam with an eye chart is important.
- A pediatric eye doctor should be seen if there is any question of visual problems.
- All children with behavior problems or learning problems should have an eye exam.

MISBEHAVING AND BUSY/STRESSED PARENTS

Both of Eddie and Kathy's parents worked long hours. "Everyone seems to get on everyone's nerves these days", their mother told me. "Both children are acting out and we are having a hard time keeping any babysitters." "When was the last time all of you had fun together," I asked? The mother frowned and said, "I don't really remember." I suggested it sounded as if the family needed some fun days now and then. Once some free days and fun were added, the children began to act like happy, normal kids.

Rx

- It is easy for a family to get caught on a treadmill.
- Children need frequent fun times with their parents.
- Picnics, riding a merry-go-round, fishing, or going to the beach or mountains are special.
- When parents and kids can't laugh together, trouble looms on the horizon.
- Every child needs daily playtime and fun time.
- If parents are caught in a work cycle, someone else needs to give the kids some fun.

TWITCHING AND LEARNING DISABILITY

A father brought in his three-year-old son because he had developed a severe movement, or tic, of his face. The child had recently lost a favorite grandfather and the parents thought that was the cause of the tic. The child had some minimal neurological signs on examination that can go along with a learning disability. An excellent educational psychologist did testing and found the child was quite severely learning disabled. The parents then remembered the tic had started when the child started preschool.

Rx

- ✓ Learning disabilities can range from mild to severe.
- ✓ A child with learning disabilities can develop school phobia.
- ✓ School phobias usually manifest at the start of a school year.
- ✓ An experienced educational psychologist needs to do testing.
- ✓ Public school testing can be limited in scope.
- ✓ Adequate testing for learning problems takes time.
- ✓ A school psychologist may not have the time or knowledge to do adequate testing.
- ✓ Learning disabilities are often passed from parent to child.
- ✓ Nervous habits may go along with learning problems.

FRUSTRATION AND HIGH EXPECTATIONS

Ted was a beautiful three-year-old who acted more like a five-year-old. His parents brought him to see me because they didn't understand his frequent outbursts of anger. I gave the child some crayons and paper to play with while his parents and I talked. He drew careful circles. "He doesn't act like a three-year-old," I said." He seems more like a five-year-old." "Neither of us has been around children", the father said. "Maybe we're expecting him to act too adult. We both bring work home and need quiet." "Yes, I said, "that could explain his anger outbursts. Ted needs to get rid of his pent-up frustration and energy."

Rx

- ✓ Expectations of a child need to be age appropriate.
- ✓ Children are not little adults.
- ✓ Happy little children are noisy.
- ✓ No little child should have to follow rigid rules of behavior.
- ✓ Kids need playtime and fun time with parents.
- ✓ Kids need lots of exercise to get rid of all their energy.
- ✓ Anger and frustration are normal emotions.
- ✓ Hiring a sitter could help if the parents need quiet times at home.

NEUROTIC AND NEEDING AFFECTION

Marla was a cute two-year-old who was often in my office with different complaints. She often would get irritable, her mother told me. The minute I came into the examining room, Marla would head for my lap and want a hug. After I finished examining Marla, the child would hold on to me, not wanting to let go. I worried about this and asked the parents to come talk with me. Both parents confessed they were not comfortable around children, even though they loved Marla. They agreed to try and give Marla more affection, which she obviously needed.

Rx

- ✓ Most kids need lots of hugs and closeness.
- ✓ Some children need more hugs than others.
- ✓ Hugs should not be conditioned on perfect behavior.
- ✓ You may not like a child's actions, but still love them.
- ✓ Life can be overwhelming for all kids at times.
- ✓ A hug can make the difference in a child's day.
- ✓ Both little boys and little girls need hugs.
- ✓ Parents may need help from a family therapist or psychologist.

MISERABLE AND EAR INFECTIONS

John was an allergic little boy who was often unhappy and frustrated. After several ear infections, his mother and father realized that when John was acting out, he usually had a medical problem, not a behavior problem. Finally, with the help of a pediatric allergist and ear, nose, and throat doctor, the ear infections stopped and John became a happy child.

Rx

- ✓ Children can have ear infections without fever.
- ✓ Little children can't localize pain or tell you.
- ✓ Tilting the head to one side can be due to an ear infection.
- ✓ Pulling or rubbing an ear can be a sign of an ear infection.
- ✓ Allergic, small children often have frequent ear infections.
- ✓ Recurrent ear infections can lead to a loss of hearing.
- ✓ A children's ear, nose, and throat M.D. should be consulted.
- ✓ Many doctors these days are not knowledgeable about ear infections and may not take the time to clear out the ear canals to be able to see a child's ear drums.

KICKING AND PARENTS DIVORCE

Tabitha never seemed like a happy child when she was in my office. A baby sitter always brought her in and I rarely saw the parents. The sitter said she kicked and screamed a lot. Eventually, the parents had an ugly divorce fighting over custody of Tabitha. The judge, after hearing the testimony of a child psychiatrist, "awarded" the little girl to her father. The child was badly scarred in the custody fight.

Rx

- ✓ Children should never be prizes given to the highest bidder or the one with the best attorney.
- ✓ A child can be destroyed by a custody fight.
- ✓ Divorced parents must put a child's interest first.
- ✓ Ongoing psychiatric care cannot always help.
- ✓ Fathers can be excellent single parents.
- ✓ If parents work together, a child can be saved.
- ✓ Keeping parents' anger away from the children is important.

HITTING AND PARENTAL GRIEVING

This little three-year-old had lost an older brother in a drowning accident. The parents constantly mourned for their lost son and found it hard to pay much attention to Rick. The child tried every possible way to get his parents' attention with daily temper tantrums, hitting, and crying spells. His parents finally realized the source of his acting out. Once they started paying attention to Rick, rather than leaving him with baby sitters, he became a different little boy.

Rx

- ✓ Losing a child can destroy a family and siblings.
- ✓ Children often think they caused a sibling's death.
- ✓ The siblings may feel great guilt they are alive.
- ✓ Talking with the siblings about the death is extremely important.
- ✓ Even little children can be aware of a terrible loss.
- ✓ Naming a child for a dead sibling can create major problems.
- ✓ Family therapy may be helpful and necessary.

HIGH STRUNG AND OVERSTIMULATION

This sweet two-year-old was brought in to see me because she seemed so high strung and nervous. In asking about the family's life style, the mother said everything was fine at home. It was only when I made a house call one day that I began to understand the problem. The house had a TV in almost every room, plus every possible kind of electronic, noisy gadget. The radio was also blaring loudly. I suspected that Caroline was a little child who needed more quiet than most kids and all the noise was causing overstimulation.

Rx

- ✓ Even little children may react strongly to loud noises.
- ✓ A constant blaring radio or TV can be upsetting to kids.
- ✓ Communication is difficult with a noisy TV or radio.
- ✓ Kids need a chance to have on-going talks with parents.
- ✓ Children with learning problems need extra quiet.
- ✓ Keeping track of how often the TV is on may help.
- ✓ Limiting TV watching can be very helpful for kids.
- ✓ Bright or creative kids may need extra quiet.

WHY CHILDREN GET UPSET AND IRRITABLE

- ✓ HUNGER
- ✓ FATIGUE
- ✓ FRUSTRATION
- ✓ EXPECTATIONS TOO HIGH
- ✓ FAMILY QUARRELING
- ✓ SPOILED
- ✓ NEEDS MORE SLEEP
- ✓ NEEDS QUIET
- ✓ NEEDS PLAYTIME
- ✓ NEEDS TIME ALONE
- ✓ UNDERLYING MEDICAL PROBLEM
- ✓ ALLERGY
- ✓ PARENTAL TENSION
- ✓ NEEDS DIAPERS CHANGED
- ✓ OVERSTIMULATED
- ✓ TOO HOT OR TOO COLD
- ✓ UNCOMFORTABLE
- ✓ NEEDS A HUG
- ✓ NEEDS REASSURANCE
- ✓ LEARNING DISABILITY
- ✓ AUTISM ASPERGERGER SYNDROME
- ✓ EMOTIONAL PROBLEM
- ✓ PARENTAL ILLNESS
- ✓ DEATH OF A SIBLING
- ✓ DEATH OF A CLOSE RELATIVE
- ✓ LITTLE TIME WITH PARENTS
- ✓ NO REGULAR ROUTINE
- ✓ NO REGULAR BEDTIME
- ✓ ANEMIC
- ✓ BORED
- ✓ REACTION TO MEDICINE
- ✓ LACK OF DISCIPLINE
- ✓ DEAF
- ✓ VISUAL PROBLEMS
- ✓ INJURY
- ✓ DIVORCE

CHECKUP LIST TO HELP PREVENT IRRITABLE TODDLERS

EATING OUT
- ✓ 1. Have you packed a small favorite toy, crayons and paper?
- ✓ 2. Have you picked a kid friendly restaurant?
- ✓ 3. Does your toddler know your rules for eating out?
- ✓ 4. If you say "No", does your child know you mean it?

BEDTIME
- ✓ 1. Have you established and do you stick to a regular bedtime for your child?
- ✓ 2. Do you have a regular routine for your child at bedtime: a bath, story, and a drink of water?
- ✓ 3. Do you allow your child to get into your bed at night?
- ✓ 4. Do you allow your child to get up and down at night?

NAPS
- ✓ 1. Does your toddler have a nap each day?
- ✓ 2. Is the nap after lunch at a regular time?
- ✓ 3. Is the house quiet when your child is napping?

OVERSTIMULATION
- ✓ 1. Is the TV on all day?
- ✓ 2. Is the radio on all day?
- ✓ 3. Does your child have a chance each day for some quiet playtime?

FEEDING

- ✓ 1. Do your fix and insist your toddler eat breakfast?
- ✓ 2. Do you include some protein in the breakfast?
- ✓ 3. Do you sit down and eat with your child?
- ✓ 4. Do you allow soft drinks or snacks between meals?
- ✓ 5. Do you limit sugary foods?
- ✓ 6. Do you give your child regular meals?
- ✓ 7. Do you rely on fast food to feed your child?

DISCIPLINE

- ✓ 1. Do you and your husband or partner discipline the same way?
- ✓ 2. Is one of you always the "heavy"?
- ✓ 3. Are you consistent with your discipline?
- ✓ 4. Are you too strict or too lenient?
- ✓ 5. Does your child understand the consequences of breaking the rules?
- ✓ 6. If you say "No", does your child know you mean it?

Section 3

PARENTING PRESCHOOLERS

INCLUDES PARENTING PRESCRIPTIONS FOR:

FEEDING TIPS 86

DISCIPLINE 87

SURVIVING
MOTHERHOOD 88

SURVIVAL TIPS
FOR FATHERS 89

SLEEP PROBLEMS 90

HANDLING FEARS 91

EMERGENCIES 92

SAFETY TIPS 93

TOILET TRAINING 94

HANDLING ANGER 95

DIVORCE 96

HIRING CHILDCARE
WORKERS 97

INFORMATION FOR
CHILDCARE WORKERS 98

FINDING A DOCTOR 99

ALLERGIES 100

GRANDPARENTS 101

DAYCARE TIPS 102

SELF-ESTEEM 103

COMMUNICATION 104

PRESCHOOL 105

HEALTH CONCERNS 106

CONSTIPATION 107

TWINS/MULTIPLE BIRTHS   108

HEALTH INSURANCE
OR AN HMO 109

FEEDING TIPS

A mother came in to talk to me because she didn't understand why meals at their house were so unpleasant. She said she tried to cook healthy foods, but her two children, ages two and four, created problems at mealtimes if she cooked anything but macaroni and cheese or things they liked. Her husband always insisted the children clean their plates and meal times were getting more and more unpleasant. "Do you have some ideas about what I can do to change things", she asked?

Rx

- ✓ Serve tempting food and don't cater to whims.
- ✓ Give single, simple foods. Kids don't like mixtures.
- ✓ Make the foods attractive.
- ✓ Give small portions.
- ✓ Ask the children to help plan healthy meals.
- ✓ Let the children plan one meal a week they would like.
- ✓ Have a child get down from the table if he or she won't eat
- ✓ Offer just juice or fruit between meals.
- ✓ Throwing food is not acceptable.
- ✓ Don't fix special meals for a child unless there are allergies.
- ✓ Use colorful plates, cups, place mats or a colorful tablecloth.
- ✓ Turn off the TV during mealtime.
- ✓ Remember a picky eater may be a picky adult eater.

SECTION 3: Parenting Preschoolers

DISCIPLINE

A mother came to my office with her preschooler almost in tears. "My husband and I can't agree on discipline" she said. He thinks children should be seen and not heard. I am his second wife and he has two grown children by another marriage. I try to shield Ray and his sister from his anger, but it seems to be getting worse and worse. If he ever hits one of the children, I will leave him. What can I do?"

I greatly feared for the marriage, but did get the father to come and talk with me. He said very strict parents had raised him and that was all he knew, but he loved his wife and children and was willing to get some help. I was greatly relieved and referred him to a male psychologist who was excellent.

Rx

- ✓ Stick to a rule when you've made it, unless it is unfair.
- ✓ Give children firm limits and structure. They need and want this.
- ✓ Don't ever spank in anger.
- ✓ Use time outs or take away privileges if discipline is needed.
- ✓ Remember discipline is love.
- ✓ At mealtimes, children should not roam around.
- ✓ Hitting or beating a child is cruel and unacceptable.
- ✓ Kids will try to manipulate you or play one parent against the other.
- ✓ Put children in their rooms without a TV, DVD player, or iPad if is discipline is needed.

SURVIVING MOTHERHOOD

I stopped into the hospital room of a new mother and found her sobbing. I knew the baby was fine because I had just checked her. Sitting next to the bed I waited until the sobbing stopped and then was horrified to have the woman tell me that her husband had just been there and said he was going to divorce her, to marry another woman! Once the mother and baby went home, I often stopped by their house in the evening to be sure everything was O.K. The woman showed great strength and was extremely grateful for my support and suggestions.

Rx

- ✓ Take time for yourself each day. Even fifteen minutes helps.
- ✓ Don't put your kids and mate's needs ahead of your own.
- ✓ Exercise daily or several times a week to reduce stress.
- ✓ Plan weekly time alone with your friends or mate. This is important.
- ✓ Take a bubble bath with the door locked and someone else watching the kids. This can be lifesaving.
- ✓ Try a new creative project: knitting, needlework, arts or crafts.
- ✓ Pay a neighborhood teenager to help daily at your busiest time.
- ✓ Vary your routine now and then to relieve stress.
- ✓ Treat yourself to something special once in a while.
- ✓ Write in a journal often to relieve stress.
- ✓ Don't skip meals. Eat lots of protein: chicken, meat, or fish.

SURVIVAL TIPS FOR FATHERS

A father was awarded custody of his three children when the mother moved out of state and abandoned the family. He desperately tried to meet all the children's needs, but this left almost no time for him. Finally, he came to see me for some help. "How can I keep up with everything", he asked? My job is suffering and I don't think the kids are happy. They miss their mother and since we don't have any nearby relatives, I am the only one to care for them." We talked about options and I suggested that hiring an older woman to live-in could be the answer. A wonderful woman was found and made the difference in the family's life

Rx

- ✓ Find a good male friend with whom you can really talk.
- ✓ Get some daily or weekly exercise. This helps a great deal.
- ✓ Have some weekly fun time away from your children.
- ✓ Don't always be the heavy in the family for discipline
- ✓ Try going to a weekly, organized fathers' support group
- ✓ Don't try to "buy" your kids with toys and gifts.
- ✓ Give your kids time not presents.
- ✓ Be sure you and your mate, if you have one, share the chores and discipline.
- ✓ Don't always be the one to get up at night with the kids or be the problem solver.

SLEEP PROBLEMS

A mother and father came to see me because they were having an on-going argument about their 4-year-old's sleeping. In the mother's culture little boys were allowed to sleep with their mothers until they started school. The father was away a lot on business trips and knew his son was sleeping with his mother during those trips. He felt this was not healthy and wanted my opinion. He said he had had talked with other fathers and they agreed. The issue had become so heated he was afraid their marriage was not going to survive. I referred him to an older woman psychologist and slowly the mother decided because her marriage was at-risk; she would not allow the little boy to sleep with her.

Rx

- ✓ Establish a regular routine at bedtime with a bath, drink, story, and toileting.
- ✓ Have a regular bedtime for each child.
- ✓ Give protein at dinnertime to help kids sleep better.
- ✓ Hang a "dream catcher" over the bed.
- ✓ Fit pajamas to the time of year.
- ✓ Put a night-light in a child's room and make the room special.
- ✓ A child should sleep in a separate room right from day one.

HANDLING FEARS

A grandmother called me saying she knew most children worried about monsters coming during the night, but since she had her grandson staying with her for several weeks, she realized his fears seems more than she would expect of most children. I asked her to bring Jed in to see me and when I examined him I saw several small tics or abnormal movements of the muscles. The little boy also seemed to be frightened and didn't want to talk. I wondered if something had happened to make him so fearful and felt he needed some professional help. A child psychiatrist discovered the child was being abused and once the abuser was put in prison, the little boy became his normal happy self.

Rx

- ✓ Talk to your child about special fears or ask him or her to draw them.
- ✓ Don't make fun of fears. This could increase them.
- ✓ Try to hide your anxiety around your children because an anxious parent makes an anxious child.
- ✓ Consult a child therapist if fears take over a child's life.
- ✓ There could be a valid reason for a fear, which needs to be discovered.
- ✓ Bath toys or bubble bath can help with a fear of bathtub water.
- ✓ Visit a firehouse, if fire engine noises are scary.
- ✓ Leave on a night-light or put stars on the ceiling that glow.
- ✓ Tape a bedtime story. A parent's voice can scare away monsters.
- ✓ An early childhood fright can leave a permanent scar if help is not received.

EMERGENCIES

I was on-call one Christmas day and had a call from parents I did not know. They said their 3-year-old was sleeping a lot and had had a fever for three days. They wanted some antibiotics, but I said I would meet them in the hospital ER, but did not give prescriptions without seeing a child. When I immediately met the family in the ER, I knew the child was in real trouble. Her color was poor, she was listless, and had a stiff neck. A spinal tap revealed thick fluid. The child had meningitis! I started an I.V., so fluids and antibiotics could be quickly given, wrote orders, talked with the parents, and sat by the child's bed to be sure she was improving. Several hours later I left for home. It was a memorable Christmas, but my teenage children entertained our guests and the child pulled though with no complications.

Rx

- Be prepared for emergencies and try not to panic. Instead use common sense.
- If a child is listless and not eating, immediate medical care must be sought.
- Know pediatric CPR as should baby sitters or daycare workers.
- Have EpiPens on hand if your child has severe allergies. A doctor or nurse could show you how to use the EpiPen. It is filled with epinephrine and can be life-saving.
- Have numbers posted by the telephone for the child's doctor, poison center, police, and fire department.
- Never let a doctor prescribe antibiotics by telephone without seeing your child.
- If your doctor is not available and you know your child is in trouble, go to the nearest hospital ER.
- You may have to be fairly assertive in an ER if they are busy and ignoring you and your child.
- Be sure all childcare people can communicate in an emergency.

SAFETY TIPS

I was at a picnic with friends near a small body of water with a small bridge over one end. Before long, I noticed a small child running onto the bridge and stopping in the middle. I didn't see any adults nearby and ran to the child. As I stood next to him, I could see two adults sitting about 200 yards away. They were paying no attention to the little boy, so I called to them and they looked over, obviously annoyed at being disturbed. I said, "If this is your child, could I bring him to you or will you come and get him? It would be very easy for him to fall into the water." The man got up slowly, giving me an unpleasant look, but did come for the child. I was relieved because I have cared for several children who drowned or were brain damaged from partially drowning. I couldn't believe the callousness of the parents.

Rx

- ✓ Empty drawers, cupboards, bedside tables and headboards of poisonous things.
- ✓ These should be locked up in a high cabinet.
- ✓ Store bleaches, polishes, and cleaners up high in a locked cabinet.
- ✓ Remove or put poisonous plants or flowers up high.
- ✓ Keep hot pots and pan handles where kids cannot reach them.
- ✓ Keep dangling electric or coffee pot cords out of a child's reach.
- ✓ Discard refrigerators, metal trunks, or big boxes with tight lids. Take these to a dump, but not anywhere kids can get into them.
- ✓ The hot water heater temperature should be below 120 degrees. Put gates at the bottom and the top of stairs to prevent accidents.
- ✓ Swimming pools, fishponds, and bodies of water can be dangerous to kids.
- ✓ Put smoke and carbon monoxide detectors in a child's room.
- ✓ Keep guns locked up securely and **unloaded.**

TOILET TRAINING

A little 3-year-old who had been easily toilet trained had a new baby sister. A few days after the baby came home, the little boy started whining and soiling his pants. His mother brought him in to see me and I found a most unhappy child. I could not find anything wrong on examination except he was constipated. After talking to the mother and seeing the beautiful little baby girl, I suspected that Timmy was not getting the attention he had always had. The parents got the constipation under control, and with some extra attention from his parents and grandparents, Timmy stopped soiling.

Rx

- ✓ Each child has his or her own age to become toilet trained. If a child is **not trained by three, a pediatrician or family doctor should be seen.**
- ✓ Use a small potty or have side rails on the big toilet.
- ✓ Be sure kids are walking and show interest before training.
- ✓ Put a child on the toilet at a regular time each day after a meal, when toilet training is started.
- ✓ Put a stool under a child's feet, if they don't touch the floor.
- ✓ Prevent a child from becoming constipated. Hard bowel movements will be difficult or painful and may be held back.
- ✓ A crack (fissure) by the anus will make it painful to have bowel movements.
- ✓ Soiling can occur around a hard, constipated bowel movement.
- ✓ If soiling occurs after a child is toilet-trained, look for constipation or an emotional problem.

HANDLING ANGER

A 3-year-old began having frequent temper tantrums and didn't want to go to preschool. After spending some time talking with the preschool teacher and several other parents, the mother decided that the little boy was just not ready for preschool and once he was allowed to stay at home or do errands with his mother, he became his old happy self.

Rx

- ✓ Ask a child to draw the anger. Talk to teachers and baby sitters about the anger.
- ✓ Children often cannot say why they are angry.
- ✓ Not every child is ready for preschool by age three.
- ✓ Plan an outing to a park or ice cream shop. There I would say "You know, I get angry sometimes and it helps me to talk about it. You seem angry. Can we talk about it?"
- ✓ Make an appointment with a children's therapist, if extreme anger persists.
- ✓ Find an art therapist, if extreme anger persists. Art therapy can be fun and helpful.
- ✓ Insist that your kids get daily exercise. This can defuse anger.
- ✓ Art, music, and fun times can help reduce anger.

DIVORCE

A divorced mother came to talk to me about her son, Tony. He had always been a happy child, but since his parents' divorce he became more and more irritable. I talked with the mother about what was going on at home and she said she had begun dating and several men had been in and out of the house. Some spent the night. I asked if there was any way she could have a college student or someone live-in, so she could spend the night with her male friends elsewhere. I said I believed that Tony was aware of the night visitors and was becoming increasingly unhappy. I also suggested a good divorce support group and gradually the mother stopped her frantic dating.

Rx

- ✓ Don't criticize the other parent or his or her family.
- ✓ Try to keep your anger away from the kids.
- ✓ Spend lots of one-to-one time with each child.
- ✓ Listen to your kids.
- ✓ Watch for signs of tension: body language and what is said.
- ✓ Arrange for some family counseling, if you need help.
- ✓ Kids want love not gifts.
- ✓ Establish limits and stick to them.
- ✓ Be consistent. If you say "No", mean it and follow through.
- ✓ Don't try buying your kids with toys, money, or gifts.

HIRING CHILDCARE WORKERS

I was always grateful to find good childcare people and found a lovely older woman to care for my 3-year-old while I was working part-time taking other doctors' practices. One day when Geoffrey was in preschool, I was working and the baby sitter was to be at the house when another mother dropped him off. I called right after he was to arrive to check that everything was O.K. Geoffrey answered the telephone and when I asked to speak to Mrs. B, he said "She isn't here." I asked how he got into the house and he replied that he had climbed in the high front window. He said he had fixed a peanut butter sandwich and was fine! I was terrified and called his nursery school teacher who lived just two houses away. She loved Geoffrey and was delighted to take him for the rest of the afternoon. It turned out that Mrs. B had confused the days.

Rx

- ✓ Check and re-check that a baby sitter knows the dates to be in charge.
- ✓ Check if the baby sitter has pediatric CPR training.
- ✓ Check the baby sitter's medical history. (Ask for a note from the applicant's physician). Obtain the date of the last TB skin test or chest X-ray.
- ✓ Security companies or Nanny agencies do background checks.
- ✓ Nanny Care is at **www.nannycare.com**
- ✓ Hire a childcare person for a trial period of one to two weeks.
- ✓ Always have a back-up plan or even two.
- ✓ Remember that letters of recommendation can be forged or written by a friend. It is safer to hire through an agency.
- ✓ Have a friend or neighbor drop by unexpectedly to check on things.
- ✓ Be sure the friend has your work and/or cell phone numbers, so you can be called, if there seems to be a problem.

INFORMATION FOR CHILDCARE WORKERS

A single parent mother forgot to refill her child's prescription for asthma medicine before she left for an over night business trip. The baby sitter called me in a panic saying the little boy was wheezing and she didn't have his usual medicine. Fortunately, my office was close to their house, so I was able to quickly care for the child. The older woman, who was baby sitting, had raised several children of her own, so knew the little boy was in trouble. She didn't have a car and not enough money for a cab and didn't think calling 911 was warranted.

℞

- ✓ **Leave all phone and cell phone numbers for a baby sitter.**
- ✓ Leave names and telephone numbers for close friends, neighbors, grandparents, and near-by relatives
- ✓ Leave numbers for your child's doctor, dentist, police, ambulance.
- ✓ Leave a list of your child's general routine, food likes, dislikes or allergies.
- ✓ List dose of any medications taken, location and time to be given.
- ✓ Check to be sure any needed medications are available.
- ✓ Show location of fire extinguishers and first-aid kit.
- ✓ Show location and instructions for thermostats or wall heaters. washer, dryer, dishwasher, and stove.
- ✓ Leave money for emergencies or needed supplies.

FINDING A DOCTOR

A mother called one day from Oregon saying her little 3-year-old had been hospitalized for mild vomiting and diarrhea without any medicine or other remedies being tried. The pediatrician was young and new in practice, so the parents knew they needed a different doctor. I researched pediatricians in their town and faxed her a list. The mother also asked what questions to ask if she had to interview several before she found one she liked.

Rx

- ✓ Ask if the doctor is part of a health plan and refers only to doctors in the HMO.
- ✓ Look at a doctor's website to check for training and board-certification.
- ✓ Ask how often the doctor is on-call at night and weekends.
- ✓ Ask who covers when the doctor is gone? Is it another pediatrician or are the patients sent to the ER. .
- ✓ Ask if the doctor sees all patients or has a nurse practitioner see some?
- ✓ Check if the doctor will meet you in the ER in emergencies. (Emergency room doctors are fine for acute trauma, but not for most pediatric problems.)
- ✓ Ask who answers questions when you call. Can you speak to the doctor when you need to?
- ✓ Ask if the doctor prescribes antibiotics over the phone or insists on seeing an ill child, as he or she should.

ALLERGIES

A little 4-year-old started complaining of pain in his head. His previous pediatrician referred him to a neurologist who ordered a CT scan of the head. It was negative. When I saw the child, he seemed pale, had dark circles under his eyes, and kept rubbing his nose. I suspected he was allergic and asked the mother to start him on an elimination diet. I also referred him to an eye doctor to have his eyes checked and to a pediatric allergist. The eye examination was negative, but the elimination diet and allergy tests showed the little boy to be highly allergic to chocolate. Once this was removed from his diet the headaches went away.

Rx

- ✓ **Have a child with serious allergies wear a Medic-Alert bracelet.**
- ✓ Alert childcare personnel, if there are serious allergies.
- ✓ Tell the parents of your child's friends about serious allergies.
- ✓ Carry and EpiPen with you at all times if there are serious allergies.
- ✓ Consult a pediatric allergist for a child who has allergies.
- ✓ Allergy-proof your house, particularly the child's room and bed.
- ✓ Many children are allergic to wool, feathers, nylon, and dust.
- ✓ Check for molds, if a child is allergic.
- ✓ Don't smoke around allergic kids, particularly asthmatic ones.
- ✓ Food allergies can be: milk, nuts, chocolate, citrus, eggs, wheat, fish.
- ✓ Watch for allergies to dogs or cats or animals with fur.
- ✓ The answer to a problem may be simple, not requiring expensive or invasive tests.

GRANDPARENTS

I was checking my new babies in the hospital nursery one morning and then visited their mothers. Most of the women were anxious to go home, but one mother asked if she could please stay two more days. I was puzzled because the nursing was going well and the mother seemed fine. Then the mother told me her mother-in-law had come to cook for her son and greatly disliked her daughter-in-law. The grandmother was leaving in two days, so I agreed the baby needed to stay two more days. The young mother was greatly relieved and when the second baby came eighteen months later, we agreed she and the baby would stay in the hospital until the mother-in-law was gone.

Rx

- ✓ Tell grandparents your rules about foods, discipline, sleeping, behavior, and gifts.
- ✓ Teach children that when grandparents are in charge their rules may be different.
- ✓ List any food allergies or intolerances.
- ✓ Try to remember grandparents on their special days.
- ✓ Don't expect grandparents to always be on-call.
- ✓ Leave your child's schedule for grandparents.
- ✓ Leave a list of all your numbers, plus child's doctor, dentist, neighbors, close friends, and especially the plumber.
- ✓ Be sure any foods, supplies, or medicines are available if the grandparents are in your home.

DAYCARE TIPS

A mother brought in her little 3-year-old for a consultation. She said Amanda was in daycare full-time because both parents worked long hours. The little girl was having frequent colds and ear infections for which the previous pediatrician kept prescribing antibiotics. The mother had to hire frequent baby sitters because the child couldn't go to daycare. When I examined Amanda, I could see thickened eardrums and suspected there was some hearing loss. A blood count showed anemia. After I referred her to a pediatric ear-nose-and throat doctor, Amanda gradually improved because the middle ears were cleaned out and tubes inserted. With treatment of the anemia, the little girl was hardly ever sick

Rx

- ✓ Ask how close is an emergency room, doctor, or hospital.
- ✓ Talk to several parents of children enrolled at the daycare center to be sure they are happy with it.
- ✓ Ask if the caretakers have yearly TB tests or chest X-rays
- ✓ Find out if the caretakers have emergency or CPR training.
- ✓ Inquire about backgrounds and references of the caretakers.
- ✓ Find out the daily routine as to naps, eating, and playtime.
- ✓ Drop in unexpectedly and see if kids are clean and happy.
- ✓ Find out if the center is licensed and the number of adults per child.
- ✓ Inquire if sick children are sent home or kept apart.
- ✓ Children can easily pick up infections in daycare if they are anemic or sick children are not sent home.

SECTION 3: Parenting Preschoolers　　　　　　　　　　　　　　　　(103)

SELF-ESTEEM

Jane, a 4-year-old was excited about starting preschool, but before long, she started crying that she wanted to stay home. The parents were puzzled, so the mother decided to visit the classroom. She soon realized the problem and later told me that that the teacher was very controlling and because Jane was quite shy, she had put her in the lowest reading group. Then she essentially ignored her. At home, Jane was reading her older brothers' books. Despite not having extra money, the parents had Jane tested for an excellent private preschool and she was accepted. There she blossomed with a wonderful teacher. From then on, she was always among the children at the top of the class.

Rx

- ✓ Find a child's special talent: music, art, dance, swimming.
- ✓ Encourage your child's positive qualities.
- ✓ A bad teacher can greatly damage a child's self-esteem.
- ✓ Give genuine praise whenever possible.
- ✓ Spend frequent one-to-one time with each child.
- ✓ Daily chores will teach responsibility and help self-esteem.
- ✓ Give lots of hugs.
- ✓ Provide counseling if a child has poor self-esteem.
- ✓ Give each child as much independence and responsibility as the age and maturity warrant.
- ✓ Arrange for outside testing by a children's educational psychologist.

COMMUNICATION

Nathan, a 4-year-old stuttered badly, but the parents had little extra money for a speech therapist. The boy became more and more angry because of his inability to communicate. The child's doctor had not suggested the parents apply for special education help, so when I saw the child that was one of the first things I did. In showing them how to get help from the special education department, Nathan was able to see a speech therapist three times a week. He soon became a different little boy once his speech began to improve and he was no longer teased.

Rx

- ✓ Spend one-to-one time with each child, as often as possible.
- ✓ Listen to your child rather than doing all of the talking.
- ✓ Watch your child's body language during conversations.
- ✓ Don't answer your cell phone when you're with your kids.
- ✓ Develop common interests with your children.
- ✓ Have meals with your children, as often as possible.
- ✓ Turn off the TV, radio, and phones during mealtime.
- ✓ When you need to discuss a problem, go for a walk, get an ice cream cone or sit in a park.
- ✓ Plan weekly special time with each child and listen.

SECTION 3: Parenting Preschoolers

PRESCHOOL

Three-year-old Graeme was to start preschool in a new town. His mother was concerned he would be afraid and took the morning off from work. This was difficult because she was in a professional training program. The little boy could hardly wait to get to school and his mother assumed she would have to stay. Instead, the boy rushed into the room and started playing with the other children. The teacher smiled and said there was no reason for the mother to stay. She couldn't believe her ears, but waved goodbye and got into her car. As she drove away, it was hard for her to realize she had an entire morning for herself!

Rx

- ✓ Tummy-aches are common if kids fear going to school
- ✓ September is the worst month for kids who fear school.
- ✓ Talk with the child's teacher if a child is unhappy at school.
- ✓ If a child is doing poorly in school have the child checked for learning, medical, or emotional problems.
- ✓ Don't be surprised that bullying happens in preschool.
- ✓ If you sense this is occurring, visit your child's class and speak with the teacher. Sometimes parents need to ban together to insist action be taken about a bully.
- ✓ Talk with the teacher if a child is unhappy at school.

HEALTH CONCERNS

The mother of an adopted 3-year-old said she knew nothing about the child's family history or any immunizations. I did a complete physical examination and asked for a urinalysis and complete blood count. Then I outlined a plan for immunizations. A tuberculin skin test was positive, so it was necessary to do a work-up for tuberculosis. The tests showed active tuberculosis, so the child was referred to a special TB clinic where excellent care was offered.

Rx

- ✓ Insist that your child have a tuberculin skin test every one to two years.
- ✓ Check that all your children's immunizations are up-to-date.
- ✓ Have a urinalysis and blood count done yearly
- ✓ Be sure the child's doctor checks his or her eyes with an eye chart each year.
- ✓ Give your child a multi-vitamin daily that your doctor suggests.
- ✓ Insist that each child have a regular bedtime.
- ✓ Ask about side effects or precautions for any medications.
- ✓ Don't give herbal medicines to kids. They can be dangerous.
- ✓ Give your kids adequate protein, vegetables, and fruits.
- ✓ Insist that your kids drink water and not many soft drinks.
- ✓ A child who drinks lots of milk and eats poorly is often anemic.
- ✓ Have a child who is frequently tired or irritable checked by the child's doctor.
- ✓ Watch that your child goes to the bathroom only 3 to 4 times a day.

CONSTIPATION

A 4-year-old was having severe problems with constipation. His pediatrician ordered a test for Celiac disease and several X-rays. These did not reveal any abnormalities other than hard bowel movements. I knew the aunt who told me the little boy and his brother lived on snacks and ate poorly at mealtime. Because the physical examination was negative except for hard rocks of stool, I asked the mother to give the little boy a stool softener and a pediatric enema. Then I wrote out a meal plan and asked her to bring the child back a few days later. It took a while to get the child eating regular meals, but once the snacks were taken away, he began to have normal bowel movements.

Rx

- ✓ Keep a three-day record of everything eaten, if a child has an on-going problem with constipation.
- ✓ Make sure adequate protein, fruits, and vegetables are eaten.
- ✓ Remove applesauce and bananas if there is constipation.
- ✓ Decrease excessive milk intake, if a child is constipated.
- ✓ Give apricot nectar and prune juice to make stools softer.
- ✓ Having a child drink lots of water will help the constipation.
- ✓ Emotional problems can cause a child to hold back bowel movements.
- ✓ A painful crack or fissure near the anus or rectum can cause bowel movements to be held back.

TWINS/MULTIPLE BIRTHS

A mother of twins said she felt isolated and was having a hard time coping. I suggested that even though money was short she needed to find a college student or teenager to help out. I suggested too, that a mothers' twin group or club would provide friends and perhaps even some baby sitting exchanges. The mother left the office in a much better mood and followed through on all my suggestions.

Rx

- ✓ Always have lots of extra baby supplies. You'll need them!
- ✓ Treat twin as a distinct personality.
- ✓ Avoid identical clothes or hairstyles.
- ✓ Provide playmates now and then.
- ✓ Join a twin parents' group or a twin online chat group.
- ✓ If you have other children, given them lots of hugs and attention.
- ✓ Look for each twin's special abilities and encourage them.
- ✓ Try to keep one twin from dominating the other one.

HEALTH INSURANCE OR AN HMO

A little boy with a progressive muscle disorder was brought in by his parents for a consultation. When I asked for the name of the child's pediatrician, so I could send a report, the parents said they didn't have one, but had a nurse practitioner. I was stunned. For a child with marked weakness and frequent lung infections, that was unbelievable. Not too long after that I was on an airplane and my seatmate turned out to be the CEO of the HMO. I told him about the little boy and he said not having a pediatrician was impossible. The man gave me his card and when the father called a few weeks later to say the child had suddenly died, I sent the CEO an email. I did not get a response.

Rx

- ✓ Check on the cost of premiums and what co-payments will be.
- ✓ Find out about restrictions and what surgeries are covered.
- ✓ Find out if prescriptions are covered partly or fully.
- ✓ Check on what hospitalizations are covered and for how many days.
- ✓ Ask if emergencies are covered elsewhere.
- ✓ Determine if any conditions are excluded from coverage.
- ✓ Find out what is covered for infants and children.
- ✓ Inquire about restrictions on seeing outside specialists.
- ✓ Ask how long the HMO has been in business and who owns it.
- ✓ Read about the appeal process if coverage is denied.
- ✓ Check on what emergencies are covered at other emergency rooms.

Section 4

PARENTING KIDS

INCLUDES PARENTING PRESCRIPTIONS FOR:

EATING 111	FINDING A DOCTOR 129
DISCIPLINE 112	ALLERGIES 130
TIPS FOR MOTHERS 113	GRANDPARENTS 132
TIPS FOR FATHERS 114	DAYCARE TIPS 133
TEACHING THE STEPS OF INDEPENDENCE 115	SELF-ESTEEM 134
EATING OUT WITH KIDS 116	COMMUNICATION 135
SLEEPING 117	TRAVELING 136
FEARS 118	TV, VIDEO GAMES AND COMPUTERS 138
EMERGENCIES 119	SCHOOL SAVVY 139
SAFETY 121	FRIENDS 140
TOILET TRAINING 123	SCHOOL PROBLEMS 141
ANGER 124	HEALTH CONCERNS 142
HANDLING DIVORCE 125	CONSTIPATION 143
EXPECTATIONS 126	SETTING AN EXAMPLE ... 144
HIRING CHILDCARE WORKERS 127	TWINS OR MULTIPLE BIRTHS 145
INFORMATION FOR CHILDCARE WORKERS 128	CHOOSING HEALTH INSURANCE OR AN HMO ... 146

SECTION 4: Parenting Kids

EATING

An anxious young mother bought her son, Sam, in for a wellness check-up. One reason for her anxiety and tenseness came out when I saw that the child had gained little weight the past year. "Sam won't eat healthy food," his mother said. "He just wants to snack and then at mealtime he is not hungry."

"What have you tried," I asked.

"Well, we all eat together like you suggested, but unless he can have exactly what he wants, such as French fries or chocolate milk; he throws a terrible temper tantrum. I'm at my wit's end. Please help me."

Rx

- ✓ Put tempting food in front of him and don't cater to his whims.
- ✓ Most children prefer single, simple foods.
- ✓ Making the food attractive and in small portions helps.
- ✓ If he doesn't eat or has a temper tantrum, have him get down from the table and stay in his room or a play area.
- ✓ Offer only juice or fruit between meals.

"He'll starve," the young mother wailed.

"No, he won't", I promised. "Call me as often as you need to, but let's see if we can make this work". On the fifth day, after a daily phone call from the distressed mother, I received the following note. *"Sam is eating us out of house and home at mealtime. What a difference it has made in our family life. He is no longer disrupting our meals."*

OTHER TIPS:

- ✓ A child who is picky about food may become an adult who is picky about food.
- ✓ Get your kids to help plan, shop, and prepare some of the meals.
- ✓ Using fun, colorful plates and cups is a good idea.
- ✓ Turning off the TV, radio, and iPhones during mealtimes allows a family to communicate and discuss problems and triumphs. This pays off richly.
- ✓ Fixing special meals, unless there are allergy problems, creates problems unless it is a birthday or other occasion.
- ✓ Cooking with spices or seasoning is usually not something kids like.

DISCIPLINE

At the monthly parents' discussion I held in my office, a six-foot-five daddy asked for help in disciplining his 4-year-old son, Rory. "He just won't listen to me", the father said. "My wife and I have read every book on discipline and tried everything suggested, but nothing works." "When you make a rule, do you both stick to it?" I asked. The father answered somewhat sheepishly, "Well, I guess not." Then I asked if Rory had ever experienced the consequences of going beyond the limits? Again, the answer was, "I guess not." "Do you and your wife discipline the same way or are you always the heavy?" The father got very thoughtful and said, "Well, I guess we've let things get out of hand. We both work and it is hard to make Rory mind when we come home tired and hungry. What can we do?" "I think," I said quietly, looking at the tall daddy, "Rory is pretty small to be in charge and it sounds as if he is running the family. I would sit down with him, go over the ground rules and the consequences of breaking them, but only if you and your wife can enforce them."

Rx

- ✓ Children need and **want** firm limits and structures.
- ✓ If you make a rule stick to it, unless you realize it is unfair and you are expecting too much.
- ✓ Discipline is love.
- ✓ Time alone for a child in his or her room, without a TV, radio, iPhone, iPad or computer is a good form of discipline. Most kids don't want to be excluded from the family conversations.
- ✓ Use time outs or take away privileges, if discipline is needed.
- ✓ Don't <u>ever</u> spank in anger.
- ✓ Encourage your kids to find healthy ways to express anger, as with: dance, art, or karate.
- ✓ A parent hitting or beating a child is <u>not</u> acceptable.
- ✓ Be careful that your kids don't try to play one parent against the other one.
- ✓ Kids are great at trying to manipulate other kids and all adults.
- ✓ At mealtimes, children should not be allowed to roam around the room.
- ✓ In public places, kids should not be allowed to scream, yell, or be disruptive.
- ✓ A child who is having a temper tantrum should be ignored, but still observed. The tantrum will usually end quickly.

TIPS FOR MOTHERS

A mother of four small children brought two of them in for physicals. As we talked, I noticed how tired and tense she appeared. *"I feel as if I am drowning"*, she said. "I have to be everything to everyone and I also help my husband in his business. The children have become whining, demanding, and I just don't know what to do."

Rx

- ✓ You need some time to be by yourself each day, so you can think, plan, or just be. Even fifteen minutes early in the morning or at night will help.
- ✓ Don't put your children's and mate's needs ahead of your own. If you do this it will create both short-term and long-term physical or emotional problems.
- ✓ Exercising daily or several times a week will help reduce your tension and stress.
- ✓ Plan weekly time alone with your mate. This is important.
- ✓ A bubble bath with the door locked and someone else watching the kids can be emotionally and physically lifesaving.
- ✓ Treat yourself to something special every so often.
- ✓ Don't skip meals, but eat lots of protein, chicken, meat, or fish, plus fruits, and vegetables.
- ✓ Watch your coffee, chocolate, and sugar intake, so it is not excessive.
- ✓ Write in a journal as often as possible. This will help relieve stress.
- ✓ A new creative project can make the days easier. Knitting, needlework, art, or crafts can all be fun.
- ✓ If possible, pay a neighborhood teenager to help daily, particularly when you are the busiest. An hour's help around dinnertime can be invaluable.
- ✓ Doing things in a different way now and then can help relieve stress. Just going window shopping or browsing in a bookstore can help. A ride on a merry-go-round can be wonderful. (I've done it alone several times.)

TIPS FOR FATHERS

A single-parent father came to see me with his children. "I need your advice," he said. "My kids seem to think I should totally devote myself to them. I don't have a life of my own. What can I do?"

My answer was I would have a family conference and let the kids know how you are feeling. Then I would ask for their suggestions about how things could be changed. "Do you really think the kids will listen and give me suggestions?" he asked. "Are they old enough to talk to like that?"

"Yes", I said "children loved to be asked for their advice and ideas even from an early age. It makes them feels important and they may have excellent suggestions".

Rx

- ✓ Making weekly one-to-one time with each of your children is important so you can get to know each other.
- ✓ Every father needs a good male friend or buddy with whom he really talks.
- ✓ Getting some daily or weekly exercise helps a great deal.
- ✓ Some weekly fun time away from your children is important to keep a balance in your life and be a person, not just a father.
- ✓ You need to treat yourself to a special CD, book, tool, or something else every now and again, since many fathers live and sacrifice for their kids.
- ✓ For fathers, it is important that you not always be the heavy in the family, where discipline is concerned.
- ✓ Some fathers enjoy a weekly, organized fathers' support group. This can be an informal get-together or one directed by a therapist.
- ✓ Don't try to "buy" your kids' love with expensive toys, gifts, or trips.
- ✓ Kids value time with a parent more than gifts, even though they may not show it or realize it.
- ✓ Discover something you and each of your children can enjoy together: reading, kite flying, woodworking, or biking.
- ✓ All fathers need to make a special effort to have time for themselves.
- ✓ Doing a new creative project by yourself can make the days better.

SECTION 4: Parenting Kids (115)

TEACHING THE STEPS OF INDEPENDENCE

A professional mother and father came to see me late one afternoon. They were good parents and I was surprised by their concern.

"We are worried because our kids seem to be such clingers. They get upset when we leave them. How can we teach them to be more independent?" they asked. As we talked about their typical day, it became apparent by hearing what the kids did and did not do that the children were having everything done for them. I suggested that a definite plan or road map needed to be developed to change this pattern.

Rx

- ✓ Kids need to have daily chores to do from early childhood, so they can learn the tools of independence.
- ✓ A chore chart is a good idea so the kids will have a definite routine to develop skills and responsibilities.
- ✓ Don't do everything for your kids, because they won't learn responsibility or develop good self-esteem.
- ✓ Each year it is important to increase a child's responsibilities. (See chore chart in the Appendix).
- ✓ Let your kids earn money rather than be given it.
- ✓ Teach both boys and girls the basics of cooking, cleaning, shopping, washing, ironing, and sewing. This will make them increasingly independent.
- ✓ As soon as possible, let your kids do jobs for adult friends you trust: baby-sitting, yard work, or running errands. This will help the kids learn about working and responsibility.
- ✓ Hire baby sitters who will let the children try to do as much as possible for themselves, rather than always doing everything for them.
- ✓ Let your kids learn to manage money. This is an important skill.
- ✓ Give praise when your kids do well.

EATING OUT WITH KIDS

I was in a nice restaurant one night seated near a family with two small children. I'm sure the kids were hungry and they were irritable. Threats were made by the parents about keeping quiet, but nothing changed and the bedlam continued. The parents were sipping glasses of wine and talking to each other, paying little attention to the children. Finally, I asked my waiter if I could move to a far corner away from the children's noise. As I ate my dinner I wondered why they would bring children to a nice restaurant if no attention is paid to them by the parents and no books, games, or crayons are brought along to keep them busy while they were waiting for food.

Rx

- ✓ Leave the children with a sitter or a friend if you aren't prepared to keep them occupied when you are in a restaurant.
- ✓ Take a favorite small toy, book, a car or doll.
- ✓ Take crayons and a small notepad.
- ✓ Take a friend for each if this isn't too expensive.
- ✓ Take a small sack with surprises to be opened every ten to fifteen minutes.
- ✓ Plan a weekly night out without your kids.
- ✓ Teach children to dress appropriately for the occasion.
- ✓ Chose a restaurant that is suitable for kids.
- ✓ Talk about what behavior you expect before you leave the house. Be sure it is age appropriate.
- ✓ Be prepared to leave the restaurant if your children don't behave.
- ✓ Eat early so the restaurant is less crowded.

SLEEPING

A mother and father came to see me looking stressed and fatigued. "We left the children home with their grandmother," they said, "because we want to talk to you. We desperately need help with our children's sleeping problems".

I wondered how the parents were able to function at all, when they explained that their 1- and 3-year-olds were up and down all night crawling in and out of the parents' bed or wanting a drink or food.

Rx

- ✓ Establish a regular routine at bedtime with a bath, drink, story, and toileting.
- ✓ Try to have a regular bedtime for each child. This is important.
- ✓ Protein at dinnertime helps kids sleep better.
- ✓ The size and kind of bed needs to fit the age.
- ✓ Soft music or a favorite story on a tape recorder may help.
- ✓ A favorite stuffed animal or dolly taken to bed can be very comforting.
- ✓ The child's room should be neither too hot nor too cold.
- ✓ A "dream catcher" over the bed can ease a child's fears. It is important to have a ritual when hanging it. Exposing it first to the sun is said to "burn away bad dreams."
- ✓ Pajamas should fit the time of year.
- ✓ A night-light can help a child sleep.
- ✓ If children are fearful about going to sleep, making their rooms special helps lessen the fears.
- ✓ You can buy stars that glow in the dark to go on the ceiling.
- ✓ Special sheets with children's characters are fun.
- ✓ Let a child pick out some special things for his or her room.
- ✓ A rocking chair in a child's room is a good place to sit for a bedtime story or to lull a little one to sleep.
- ✓ Mommy or daddy's voice coming out of a tape recorder telling a favorite story or reading favorite poems may help a child go to sleep.
- ✓ A noisy TV, radio, or loud talking in other rooms can keep a child awake.
- ✓ Frequent bad dreams or nightmares should be investigated by a physician or children's therapist.
- ✓ Cokes or caffeine containing drinks can cause sleeplessness.

FEARS

A mother called one afternoon and said that she had a quick question. "What can I do about my 3-year-old's multiple fears? He is afraid of the vacuum, water, loud noises and many other things." I replied that it would be best to see the child and then we could talk afterwards. When the little boy came in with his mother, he seemed anxious and overactive. Slowly the story came out that the mother-in-law lived with the family and there was a great deal of friction between her and Roy's mother. The grandmother was always buying treats for Roy and spoiled him badly. Roy was being pulled between his mother and grandmother and I suspected his fears were symptoms of underlying anxiety.

My advice was for the boy to see a child therapist who specialized in play therapy. (Play therapy is where a child uses dolls to act out family interactions. It can be very helpful in understanding family dynamics.) I also urged the parents to consider some counseling although I suspected this wouldn't happen. Unfortunately, the couple's problems ended in divorce, but at least the little boy did get some on-going help from a child therapist.

Rx

- ✓ Don't make fun of fears because this could increase them.
- ✓ Talk to your child about any special fears or ask him or her to draw them.
- ✓ Try to hide your anxiety around your children because an anxious parent makes an anxious child.
- ✓ Consult a child therapist if fears take over one of your children's lives.
- ✓ Buy inexpensive bath toys, if there is a fear of bathtub water. Bubbles can help too.
- ✓ Visit a firehouse, if fire engine noises are scary.
- ✓ Leave a light on or have little stars on the ceiling, to help decrease nighttime fears.
- ✓ Tape a bedtime story because a parent's voice coming from a bedside tape recorder can scare monsters away.
- ✓ Buy or have a child make his or her own Native American "dream catcher" to catch bad dreams. Make a ceremony of putting up the dream catcher.
- ✓ Exposing the dream catcher to the sun is said to burn away bad dreams.

SECTION 4: Parenting Kids

EMERGENCIES

A mother called one night just as I was leaving my office saying that her son, Sam, had fallen with a stick in his mouth. "It's bleeding," she said, "but I think it's okay. Maybe I'll bring him in tomorrow and have you look at it." No", I said, "If something needs to be done, we should not wait until tomorrow. Please bring him in right now." It took a little urging, but the mother arrived about thirty minutes later. Sam was still crying, but with a little coaxing, I was able to see the roof of his mouth where there was a large gaping hole. I quickly called an excellent surgeon and the hole was repaired that evening. I was glad that I had insisted on seeing the child. In emergencies, the old adage does pay off; "it's better to be safe than sorry" and "a stitch in time can often save more in the future."

Rx

- ✓ Be prepared for emergencies and try not to panic, but use your common sense.
- ✓ Know pediatric CPR and be sure that your baby sitter and daycare workers know it.
- ✓ Have a bee sting kit, if bee allergies are a problem in your family.
- ✓ Have EpiPens on hand if your child has severe allergies. (Your doctor or allergist should show you how to use the EpiPen syringe which is filled with epinephrine and can be life-saving.)
- ✓ Have numbers posted by the telephone for the child's doctor, poison center, police, and fire department.
- ✓ Be sure all baby sitters or childcare people are able to communicate with emergency personnel.

REAL EMERGENCIES ARE:

- ✓ Severe, uncontrolled bleeding.
- ✓ Choking on a foreign object, such as a peanut or hard candy.
- ✓ Severe asthma attack with inability to pass air in or out.
- ✓ Stiff neck with fever and headache.
- ✓ Convulsion or seizure.
- ✓ Drug or poison ingestion.
- ✓ Severe allergic reaction to bees or food.
- ✓ Loss of consciousness.
- ✓ Fracture of arm, leg, or any serious break.
- ✓ Severe or prolonged vomiting or diarrhea.
- ✓ Severe burns.
- ✓ Any eye injury.
- ✓ Difficulty breathing.
- ✓ High, prolonged fevers.
- ✓ Severe croup.
- ✓ Rapidly progressive unusual skin rashes or blotches.
- ✓ Gun shot wound.

SECTION 4: Parenting Kids

SAFETY

A distraught parent called one day from work saying that her little boy had wandered into his grandmother's bedroom and swallowed several of her heart pills from the nightstand. He thought they were candy. I asked that the grandmother rush him to the emergency room because the pills could be dangerous for a 3-year-old to ingest. I met the child and his grandmother in the ER and pumped the child's stomach. Then, I kept him there for several hours' observation.

Rx

- ✓ All drawers, cupboards, bedside tables and headboards need to be emptied of poisonous things. Then these should be locked up or put in a high cabinet.
- ✓ Bleaches, polishes, and cleaners should be stored high up or in a locked cabinet.
- ✓ Put poisonous plants or flowers up high or in a room where a child is not allowed.
- ✓ Keep hot pots and pan handles where kids can not reach them.
- ✓ Keep dangling electric or coffee pot cords out of a child's reach.
- ✓ Old refrigerators, metal trunks, or big boxes with tight lids should be discarded in a dump or not left anywhere kids can get into them.
- ✓ Check the temperature of your hot water heater to be sure it is below 120 degrees.
- ✓ Gates at the bottom and the top of stairs will prevent accidents.
- ✓ Check to be sure that you have adequate and functional smoke and carbon monoxide detectors. (Carbon monoxide poisoning can occur from wall heaters and other sources.)
- ✓ Keep guns unloaded and locked up securely.
- ✓ Teach children the three rules regarding fires: **stop – drop – roll.**
- ✓ Always insist that helmets be used for bike riding, skiing, and skateboarding.
- ✓ A child's name visible on a bag or barrette will let a stranger be able to call the child's name, thus appearing to be a friend, so the child will go with him.
- ✓ Teach children that the washing machine and clothes dryer are off limits.
- ✓ Have children learn to swim early.

- ✓ Teach your kids a password an unfamiliar adult must use if he or she says there is an emergency and the individual is to take them to their parents.
- ✓ Place grandmothers' or visitors purses up high. They may contain medicines.
- ✓ Talk about safety rules and have emergency fire drills.
- ✓ Teach children to use a fire extinguisher or rugs to put out small fires.
- ✓ Always have a responsible adult present in the house.
- ✓ Place fire extinguishers in strategic places.
- ✓ Check your smoke detectors twice yearly.
- ✓ Protect kids from falling into swimming pools by having high fences or specially designed covers. (Be sure a child is not able to slip under a pool cover or it could close up around them.)
- ✓ Have locks up high on outdoor gates.
- ✓ Clean up after a party, particularly if glasses on low tables contain left-over alcohol or cigarette butts are accessible.

TOILET TRAINING

The mother of a child who had spina bifida told me her other child had been toilet trained, but had recently started soiling. When I examined the child and did a rectal examination, I found hard stool in the rectum. I suspected the little girl was resenting all the attention being paid to her older sister. Once she received more attention and the constipation was under control, the soiling ceased.

Rx

Each child has his or her own age to become toilet trained. If a child is not trained by about three, then a pediatrician or family doctor should be seen. There are rectal and bowel problems that make toilet training difficult.

- ✓ Making a big fuss about a child not being toilet trained will make things worse. It will happen in time, unless there are medical problems.
- ✓ Use a small potty or have side rails on the big toilet, so that a child feels secure.
- ✓ Kids usually don't become toilet trained until they can walk and also show interest in becoming trained.
- ✓ When you start toilet training, put a child on the toilet at a regular time each day after a meal.
- ✓ Put a stool under a child's feet if they don't touch the floor when he or she is sitting on the big toilet.
- ✓ Prevent a child from becoming constipated because the bowel movements will be difficult or painful and held back.
- ✓ Teach your children that the toilet is not for play or for washing a little sibling's hair, as did one older brother when his mother was ill in bed.

IMPORTANT THINGS TO REMEMBER:

- ✓ A crack or fissure at the edge of the rectum (anus) may keep a child from having a bowel movement because of the pain.
- ✓ Some kids normally have a bowel movement just every two or three days.
- ✓ The color of a bowel movement can be altered by food or drink such as Kool-Aid.
- ✓ Small toilet seats are convenient for traveling with small children. They fit on top of a regular toilet seat.

ANGER

A tired young mother of four children came to see me. "I just brought two children for their exams," she said, because later, if the children can wait in the playroom, I would like talk to you about Steven. I don't know what to do with him. He always seems so angry. The other day I looked at him and realized that I hadn't seen him laugh or be happy in a long, long time. Also he has temper outbursts if things don't go his way."

"Have you asked him why he is angry," I asked?

"But," his mother said, "He's only five. Can you really talk to a 5-year-old?"

"Yes", I said and made some suggestions.

Remember than angry, unhappy children may become angry, unhappy adults.

Rx

- ✓ Plan an outing to a park or to an ice cream shop where it is quiet and you can talk. Sitting across from each other, I would say, "You know, I get very angry sometimes and don't know why but it helps to talk to someone. I have noticed that recently you seem angry. Can we talk about it?"
- ✓ Ask a child to draw what causes the anger.
- ✓ Make an appointment with a trained children's therapist for play therapy if excessive anger persists.
- ✓ Look for an art therapist if extreme anger persists. Art therapy can also be very helpful and fun if the art therapist is trained to work with children.
- ✓ Talk to teachers and baby sitters about a child's anger. This may give some insight to the anger. A learning disability could be present that would need professional testing to detect.
- ✓ Insist that your kids get some daily exercise because this can help defuse anger.
- ✓ Provide karate lessons if possible for kids with considerable anger.
- ✓ Look for a child's special talents or abilities and encourage these. This can help get rid of anger.
- ✓ Keep your own anger outbursts under control, if possible, because a child may model angry outbursts after a parent.

HANDLING DIVORCE

A recently divorced mother talked to me about her 4-year-old child "My son doesn't want me out of his sight, she said, "I knew the parents had been through a bitter divorce and the father was recently remarried. I told the mother it would take time for Joe to adjust to the new situation. Children need to feel safe and secure and the boy probably needed lots of reassurance. He could feel that his mother was also going to leave. A few visits with a wonderful child psychologist helped Joe feel more secure so he could allow his mother out of his sight.

For other parents in similar situations, I would ask:

- ✓ Do you and his father try to keep your anger away from your kids or do you tear each other down? This can be very destructive for kids.
- ✓ Do your children feel as if both parents might leave? Most kids will have this fear.
- ✓ Has either parent started dating or is a stranger spending nights in the house? This can give children a feeling of insecurity, particularly if there is a frequent turnover.

Rx

- ✓ Don't criticize the other parent or his or her family.
- ✓ Spend lots of one-to-one time with each child.
- ✓ Listen to your kids.
- ✓ Watch for signs of tension in your kids. Watch body language, as well as what is said. Clues about tension, anger, or fear can be picked up by careful observation.
- ✓ Talk about anger and ways it can be handled or the ways you handle your own anger. (I pull weeds I've labeled with someone's name or hit a tennis ball.)
- ✓ Arrange for some family counseling, if you need help in handling anger.
- ✓ Establish limits and keep them even though they may be different in mother's or father's house. Kids can adapt to rules, if they know what they are.
- ✓ Be consistent. If you say **"No"**, mean it and follow through.
- ✓ Don't try buying your kids with toys, money, or gifts. They want love and time, not toys or gifts.

EXPECTATIONS

"Our child, Kevin, has not been accepted at the private school we want and his father is livid," a mother said. The school suggested some special professional help for our son but neither of us think is necessary and we would like your opinion."

After a thorough history and examination, I suspected a learning disability and suggested that my favorite educational psychologist do some testing. A rather marked learning disability was found, which the parents wouldn't accept. "With tutoring," I said, "Your son should be able to do well." Unfortunately, the father and mother, both successful professionals, found this unacceptable. They sought another opinion.

Your dreams for your child may not and probably will not be the dreams the child will have for himself or herself.

Expectations must reflect the time, the place, and the child's abilities.

A child should be allowed to have and pursue his or her own dreams.

Rx

- ✓ Plan some daily time and have lives of your own, as parents.
- ✓ Evaluate expectations periodically and change if necessary.
- ✓ Insist that conversations on and off the telephone are possible without kids demanding attention.
- ✓ Expect children to behave if you re eating out.
- ✓ Don't center all the day's activities around the children. Kids need to learn how to amuse themselves.
- ✓ Plan activities to occupy kids if they have to sit still for a long period.
- ✓ Allow kids to have some say in how they dress, but if what they want to wear is unacceptable to you, say so. (They don't want to be embarrassed by the way you dress, so it should work both ways.)

HIRING CHILDCARE WORKERS

In the small affluent town of La Jolla, California I found one to two children a year to have positive tuberculin skin tests. Further testing showed they had active TB. Sometimes a grandparent was the one found to have exposed the child to tuberculosis, but usually it was the baby sitter or childcare person. The parents had not asked about the caretaker's most recent chest X-ray or tuberculin test, when he or she was hired. This is extremely important now that some of the TB bugs are quite resistant to medication. TB tests or chest X-rays can be obtained at no cost at most health departments.

Rx

- ✓ Check if the baby sitter has pediatric CPR training.
- ✓ Check the baby sitter's medical history. (You can ask for a note from the applicant's physician). Obtain the date of the last tuberculin skin test or chest X-ray.
- ✓ Hire a childcare person for a trial period of one to two weeks. Have a friend or neighbor drop by unexpectedly and check on things. Be sure the friend has your work and/or cell phone numbers, so your can be called, if there seems to be a problem.
- ✓ Let children who are old enough and interested help interview prospective child-care people.

Remember that letters of recommendation from a previous employer can be forged or written by a friend. It is safest to hire through a recognized, licensed agency, such as Nannycare.

INFORMATION FOR CHILDCARE WORKERS

A baby sitter called me late one afternoon saying that the 4-year-old, Johnny, was ill and having trouble breathing. The parents were off skiing in Colorado and the baby sitter didn't drive. I was worried after the call and was at the home within thirty minutes. It was good that I did because the little boy was gray and breathing with difficulty. I suspected Johnny had pneumonia, which was later confirmed by a chest X-ray. I immediately arranged for a hospital admission and drove the child to the hospital where we put him in an oxygen tent. The parents had left a telephone number where they could be reached, but apparently changed hotels or were visiting friends. It was a scary seven days before the child recovered and I was able to take him home.

Rx

- Leave all your phone and pager numbers for a baby sitter.
- Leave current telephone numbers for: close friends, grandparents, and any near-by relatives. neighbors' names and telephones numbers. the doctor, dentist, police, fire department, and ambulance.
- Leave a list of your child's general routine.
- Leave a list of scheduled activities, if there are any, with time, dates, and addresses.
- Make a list of your child's food likes and dislikes and any allergies.
- List any medications taken; the dose, their location, plus the time to be given.
- Note or show location of fire extinguishers.
- Note or show location and instructions for the furnace thermostat or wall heaters.
- Leave written instructions about the washer, dryer, dishwasher, and stove.
- Post or show the location of the first aid kit.
- Be sure the baby sitter can communicate if there is an emergency.
- Leave money for emergencies, particularly for a prolonged absence.

SECTION 4: Parenting Kids (129)

FINDING A DOCTOR

A former patient called one day from New York City asking if I could help find a new pediatrician for her children. She had had bad experiences with two different ones, she said. One was never in his office and the other one was abrupt and often unavailable. She asked what questions to ask to check out a new doctor. I did some research about doctors in her vicinity and had the following questions faxed to her.

Rx

- ✓ Ask if the doctor is part of a health plan and refers only to doctors in the HMO.
- ✓ Find out how often the doctor is on-call at night and weekends and who covers when he or she is gone? Check if another pediatrician sees the children or if they are seen by ancillary medical personnel.
- ✓ Check whether the doctor will meet you in the ER for emergencies or instead has the ER doctor see your child? (Emergency room doctors are fine for acute trauma but not for most pediatric problems.)
- ✓ Ask who answers questions when you call and can you speak to the doctor when you need to. You might not be told the truth about this and may have to learn the hard way.
- ✓ Inquire if the doctor prescribes antibiotics over the phone or instead insists on seeing an ill child. Kids must be examined before antibiotics are prescribed because a serious illness can be missed.
- ✓ Ask if he or she has one or more offices and if so find out how many days a week is he or she in each one. A second office could be at a great distance that would not work for you.
- ✓ Check on the fees for routine and other visits and if the office staff will bill insurance companies.
- ✓ Find out about the doctor's credentials. Is he or she an M.D. or D.O?
- ✓ Inquire if the doctor is board certified in his or her specialty. (This means specific tests have been passed after the training requirements are completed.)
- ✓ Ask how close the doctor's office is to a hospital and what hospital he or she uses.
- ✓ In an emergency, it is important that a doctor can arrive quickly at the hospital.
- ✓ Find out how much time the doctor allots to each patient.
- ✓ Ask how close the doctor's office is to your house or where your child is in school or childcare.
- ✓ Visit the office to check if it is clean and pleasant.
- ✓ See if the office staff members are pleasant and helpful.

ALLERGIES

I had an unforgettable call one day about Tommy, a little boy who had been stung by a bee. He was having trouble breathing and I immediately met the mother and child in the local emergency room. Fortunately, the reaction was treatable with benadryl and epinephrine. Previously, I had advised the mother to buy a bee sting kit, which she had done and our office nurse had shown her how to use the epinephrine-filled syringe which was in the kit. The mother was too frightened to inject the epinephrine, which could have been fatal for Tommy. (Epinephrine can be lifesaving and the syringe in the bee sting kit is easy to use. Now that EpiPen is available as a syringe containing epinephrine, it is easier to use.)

Rx

- ✓ Order a Medic-Alert bracelet for a child with serious allergies and insist it is always worn.
- ✓ Alert childcare and school personnel if there are serious allergies.
- ✓ Tell the parents of your child's friends if there are serious allergies.
- ✓ Carry an EpiPen with you at all times, if a child has serious allergies.
- ✓ Consult a pediatric allergist for a child who has allergies and then see the doctor as needed.
- ✓ Allergy-proof your house, particularly the child's room and bed. Many children are allergic to wool, feathers, and some even to nylon. Check what mattresses and pillows contain. Dust can be a major problem in heavy drapes or any other dust catchers.
- ✓ Don't smoke around allergic children, particularly those with asthma.
- ✓ Check for molds if a child is allergic.
- ✓ Watch for food allergies, as milk, nuts, chocolate, citrus, eggs, fish, and wheat.
- ✓ Some children are allergic to soy.
- ✓ Watch for allergies to dogs or cats or animals with fur.
- ✓ Be careful about latex products around some allergic kids and children with spina bifida.
- ✓ Check that cleaning products and soaps are not allergenic.

SIGNS OF ALLERGY CAN BE:

- ✓ Frequent colds or ear infections.
- ✓ Dark circles under the eyes.
- ✓ Rubbing the nose frequently, called an "allergic salute".
- ✓ Diarrhea that could be due to milk intolerance.
- ✓ Sneezing frequently.
- ✓ A constant runny nose.
- ✓ Wheezing or difficulty breathing.

GRANDPARENTS

A worried father brought in his 2-month-old, Taylor because he thought the baby was not gaining enough weight. The baby was fine, but as I listened I suspected that the father wanted to talk to me about something else. It turned out that he was very worried about his wife and the way she and his mother were interacting. The grandmother had come to help, but many problems were arising. She was from Africa and the way she insisted things be done was not what the baby's mother had learned from books and parenting classes. I wrote out detailed instruction for the mother and urged the parents to call if they needed support or wanted me to make a house call. I did visit the home and was able to speak with the grandmother. The mother told me later that this helped considerably.

Rx

- ✓ Treasure grandparents, but let them know that the kids are yours – not theirs.
- ✓ Tell grandparents the rules you want enforced about foods, discipline, sleeping, behavior, and gifts.
- ✓ Teach children to respect their grandparents.
- ✓ Teach children that when they are with their grandparents the grandparents are in charge and their rules may be different.
- ✓ Don't expect grandparents to always be on call as baby sitters. They need a life of their own.
- ✓ Give or send a gift or flowers now and then to say thank you to grandparents for baby sitting. It will be greatly appreciated.
- ✓ Send valentines when you can on Valentine's Day, particularly if a grandparent is alone.
- ✓ Celebrate grandparent's birthdays or send birthday cards your kids can make.
- ✓ Try to remember grandparents' special days, such as anniversaries.
- ✓ Be aware of medical or physical problems grandparents may have. These could limit their ability to baby-sit.
- ✓ Leave an up-to-date list of numbers for the: cell phones, work phones, child's doctor, dentist, near-by neighbors, close friends, household help, and especially the plumber.
- ✓ Ask your child's doctor or the grandparent's doctor for help, if you are having a problem with a grandparent.
- ✓ Leave your baby's schedule for the grandparents, if they are baby-sitting. List any food allergies or food intolerances.

SECTION 4: Parenting Kids

DAYCARE TIPS

A distraught parent called one day from work saying that her little boy, Ben, had wandered into a neighbor's back yard from his daycare and swallowed something in an open coke bottle. The daycare people were frantic and didn't know what to do.

I met the mother at the emergency room and did not pump the child's stomach because I could see burns in the child' mouth. It turned out that the detergent had burned the tube to the stomach or esophagus and it took many surgeries for Ben to be able to swallow again.

Rx

- ✓ Talk to several parents of children enrolled in a daycare program prior to enrolling your child to see how they would rate it.
- ✓ Ask about the number of children for each adult caretaker.
- ✓ Check on the policy about illness. Is an ill child sent home or kept away from the well children?
- ✓ Drop in unexpectedly.
- ✓ Inquire if a daycare center is licensed.
- ✓ Ask how close is an emergency room, doctor, or hospital.
- ✓ Check on the training of the caretakers.
- ✓ Find out if any of the caretakers have emergency training, as pediatric CPR.
- ✓ Look to see if the daycare center is clean.
- ✓ Visit to see if the children seem happy and not overly controlled.
- ✓ Ask if the caretakers are required to have yearly TB tests or chest X-rays.
- ✓ Inquire if the backgrounds and references of the caretakers are thoroughly checked.
- ✓ Find out the daily routine as to naps, eating, and playtime.
- ✓ Look to see if there is a warm, comfortable place for little children to nap.
- ✓ Ask how long the daycare has been in business.
- ✓ Inquire if the children are served any hot food.
- ✓ Look to see if the cleaning and dishwashing supplies are kept up high.

SELF-ESTEEM

A mother and father came to see me about their 6-year-old Laurie's extreme shyness. In talking to them, as well as my past knowledge of the family, I knew that achievement was all-important to these parents. Laurie was poorly coordinated and disliked sports. This was unfortunate because sports were important to both parents.

"Perhaps Laurie feels she can't live up to your expectations," I said. "I would look for and encourage some other special ability of hers. That way she will have something she can do well". The parents became thoughtful and promised that they would try. These good parents enrolled Laurie in a child's art class, where she excelled and which she loved.

Rx

- ✓ Find and help develop a child's special talent: music, art, dance, poetry, swimming.
- ✓ Always stress your child's positive qualities.
- ✓ Give lots of hugs.
- ✓ Praise your child, but only when warranted.
- ✓ Spend one-to-one fun time with each of your children, as often as possible.
- ✓ Plan daily chores to teach responsibility and develop self-esteem.
- ✓ Let each child earn part of the money you give.
- ✓ If a learning problem is suspected, arrange for outside testing by a children's educational psychologist.
- ✓ Provide counseling if a child has poor self-esteem.
- ✓ Keep a scrapbook for each child to remember special events or achievements.
- ✓ Give each child as much independence and responsibility, as the age and maturity warrant.

SECTION 4: Parenting Kids

COMMUNICATION

A little boy seemed to be withdrawing more and more from his parents and was never happy. His silence was extremely worrisome, so the father brought the child in to see me. As we talked, I sensed a tense, unhappy little boy, but could find no medical reason for this. When the father told me that both he and his wife had to travel for their jobs a great deal, I wondered if this wasn't part of the problem. I asked about the baby sitter and if there were close friends, involved grandparents, or friendly neighbors. Apparently, the family was new to the area and their house was quite isolated. Slowly, I began to see a picture of a lonely little boy who needed much more time with his parents. Eventually, the parents were able to change their jobs, so they were at home more. The little boy became his old happy self to everyone's delight.

Rx
_____

- ✓ Spend one-to-one time with each child, as often as possible.
- ✓ Listen to your child rather than doing all of the talking.
- ✓ Watch your child's body language during conversations.
- ✓ Put your cell phone away. Don't answer it when you're with your kids.
- ✓ Develop common interests with your children, as reading, biking, or swimming.
- ✓ Have meals with your children as often as possible and listen to them.
- ✓ Turn off the TV, radio, and phones during mealtime.
- ✓ Set the stage when you need to talk about a problem. Go for a walk, get an ice cream cone, or sit on a park bench together.
- ✓ Plan a weekly get-together with each child to keep communication open.
- ✓ Talk about a problem you have had to see if this will get some dialogue started.
- ✓ Ask a child for his or her advice about a situation or problem that would be within their reality.
- ** *If none of these ideas are successful then I would suggest some therapy for a child with whom you are having communication problems.*

TRAVELING

A family was coming home from a reunion in the Chicago area. Suddenly, their son, Ken, became ill, so they rushed him to a nearby urgent care center. The doctor did some tests and said Ken had diabetes. The parents were uncomfortable with this diagnosis and instead drove all night. They were at my office first thing the next morning and I found that Ken had pneumonia, not diabetes. With some antibiotics, he slowly recovered.

Rx

TRAVELING BY CAR

- ✓ Make sure you have approved car seats for small children or if the kids are older insist they put on their seatbelts.
- ✓ Be sure you have adequate supplies for your children, in case car trouble develops. This would include water, snacks, and any medications that are being taken.
- ✓ Carry lots of Wash N' Dries or HandiWipes in your car.
- ✓ Make room for a favorite toy, doll, blanket, or pillow.
- ✓ Insist that your children behave. Accidents can happen if the driver gets distracted settling fights in the back seat.
- ✓ Take along a deck of cards.
- ✓ Have small protein snacks tucked in your travel bag.
- ✓ Play a license plate game looking for as many states as possible, if the children are old enough.
- ✓ Take small, magnetic travel games for older children
- ✓ Tuck lots of small surprises in your travel bag.
- ✓ Play games such as "I Spy" to look for logos, letters, or words, to keep children occupied.
- ✓ Avoid hard candy and nuts which kids can choke on. These are particularly dangerous when traveling in a car. You may be driving at high speed on a busy freeway and can't safely stop to help.
- ✓ Have juice or water readily available.

SECTION 4: Parenting Kids

- ✓ Take a first aid kit.
- ✓ Make frequent stops, so the kids can get out and move around.

TRAVELING BY AIRPLANE

- ✓ Talk about the trip ahead of time and tell your kids what is expected of them.
- ✓ Have your children swallowing or chewing when the plane takes off or lands in order to open their ear (Eustachian) tubes.
- ✓ Insist that your kids behave.
- ✓ Have some small surprises that you can pull out periodically to keep the children occupied.
- ✓ Let each child take a favorite toy, doll, blanket, pillow, book, or DVD.
- ✓ Take along a deck of cards.
- ✓ Take along small, magnetic travel games. These can be fun.

TV, VIDEO GAMES AND COMPUTERS

A bright 6-year-old boy, Roger, came in for his physical examination. In answer to the question about how much time he spent watching TV or playing video games, his mother said, "Well, he doesn't have any friends close by and since both my husband work, I'm afraid the baby sitter lets him watch too much TV."

Roger was a thin, unhappy appearing little boy who wore glasses and seemed ill at ease. He wouldn't make eye contact, which alarmed me. (Lack of eye contact is an important sign and can indicate a problem.) I asked the nurse to take Roger to the playroom for a little while, so I could talk to his mother alone. We discussed how Roger could play more with other kids and not watch so much TV. After talking about various possibilities, the mother worked out a way the boy could be in an after-school recreation program. A few months later, a much happier boy came to my office.

Rx

- ✓ Don't allow your child's world to be dominated by machines of any kind: TV, video games, computers, iPads, or DVDs. Be sure a child has plenty of interaction with other children and adults.
- ✓ Prevent a child, who has a TV or a computer in his or her own room, from becoming isolated. It is difficult to monitor what is being watched or accessed on the computer.
- ✓ Keep track of how much daily time the kids watch TV.
- ✓ Monitor what your kids watch on T.V.
- ✓ Be aware of what your kids are doing on the computer, as to chat rooms, texting and Websites.
- ✓ Be as knowledgeable about the computer as your kids. It is hard!
- ✓ Keep track of how much time your child uses the computer or plays video games and don't allow excessive use.
- ✓ Block sites that kids should not view if your kids are accessing them.
- ✓ Insist that your kids play with friends as often as possible.
- ✓ Get your kids to play outdoors when the weather is good. Provide, if possible, games such as shuffleboard, horseshoes, badminton, or a basketball hoop. These can be incentives to play outside.

SCHOOL SAVVY

A school principal, as well as the boy's teacher, refused to admit that Ryan needed special help. Fortunately, the parents were able to pay for outside testing by a children's educational psychologist who found a marked learning disability. The principal and school psychologist refused to accept the testing, so the parents hired a special education attorney. They knew their child better than the school personnel and insisted that Ryan get the help he needed. They battled hard to get him special education help, but said it was worth all the time and money they spent.

Rx

- ✓ Get to know the school principal and secretary by name.
- ✓ Give school staff your telephone and pager numbers, as well as those of relatives and your child's doctor if you are not available.
- ✓ Get to know your child's teachers.
- ✓ Speak up about the amount of homework your child has if it seems overwhelming or if your child seems bored and needs some special projects. School should be interesting and stimulating.
- ✓ Check out the school rules about who picks up a child and if the rules are enforced.
- ✓ Visit your child's class now and then, but call ahead of time.
- ✓ Attend school performances whenever you can.
- ✓ Volunteer your time if you can.
- ✓ **Don't expect the school to do your parenting.**
- ✓ Get to know your child's friends and their parents.
- ✓ Find out how to get necessary testing and help if you suspect your child has a learning disability. Other parents can be very helpful and special education attorneys are available in many cities.
- ✓ Be as involved as possible in the school parents' group or PTA.
- ✓ Get to know the school board members and vote in local elections.
- ✓ Become acquainted with the bus driver or drivers and be sure the buses are well maintained.
- ✓ Donate time, books, or money to the school library, if you can.

FRIENDS

A young mother said one day in my office. "I am amazed or rather horrified at the amount of money parents spend in this town on lavish birthday parties and clothes. We can't spend that kind of money and don't want our kids to think that money grows on trees. What can we do?"

Rx

- ✓ Invite some parents of your child's friends over to discuss expensive birthday parties, sleepovers, money spent for clothes, etc.
- ✓ Be sure the parents of your child's friends have all your telephone numbers.
- ✓ Be sure the parents of your kids' friends are reliable about picking up and delivering your children on time.
- ✓ Find out if the parents of your children's friends pretty much agree with your views on safety, drinking, driving, and dressing.
- ✓ Always meet the parents of your children's friends.
- ✓ Be sure the parents of your children's friends are physically present when your kids are at their homes.
- ✓ Be sure the homes where your children visit have any guns unloaded and under lock and key.

SCHOOL PROBLEMS

A very bright five year old, Rory, was excited about starting kindergarten. He had not gone to preschool because the family was overseas and there were no preschools. As the summer was ending, the little boy questioned his mother each day about how long it would be until school started. Finally the BIG day arrived and Rory ran pell-mell into the school while his mother hurried to keep up. At the end of the morning, Rory's mother couldn't believe her eyes when she picked up her son. The little boy was waiting for her by his classroom door, looking very dejected. "What happened", the worried mother asked? "I didn't learn to read today", Rory said, "You said I would learn to read in kindergarten!"

Rx

- ✓ Try to remember your first day of school and think about how each of your children will react. Some will be shy, others excited, and some will feel terror.
- ✓ Be aware that tummy-aches are very common in children who fear going to school. Other physical symptoms may develop in kids who are unhappy about a teacher, class, or those who have trouble learning.
- ✓ September is the worst month for kids who fear a new teacher, new classmates, and often a new school.
- ✓ Don't be surprised that bullying can happen even in nursery school or preschool. If you sense this is occurring, visit your child's classroom and speak with the teacher. Sometimes several parents need to ban together to insist something be done about a bully.
- ✓ Talking about how to handle a bully with your children or children is important. Some karate or other lessons may be needed.
- ✓ Talk with the teacher if a child is over-burdened with homework.
- ✓ Have a bright child, who is doing poorly in school, checked by a professional to see if there are learning, medical, or emotional problems. Testing for a learning problem should be done by an experienced, educational child psychologist, preferably one not employed by the schools.
- ✓ Check that intense pressure to perform in sports is not being applied to kids. Even little children may be under pressure to excel in sports.
- ✓ Fun and exercise should be the object of games and sports, not winning. Undue pressure by the school personnel or parents can cause havoc with kids.
- ✓ Talk with your child if your child's teacher or principal complain he or she is bullying other kids. Professional help may be needed.

HEALTH CONCERNS

A newly widowed father brought his children to my office for the first time. He was planning a trip to Mexico and wanted to be sure that he took the proper supplies and medicines for his kids. In going over their medical histories, the father had little information about past immunizations and the kids did not remember any shots. I persuaded the father to delay the trip to Mexico until the children's immunizations were at least partly completed. I had real fears that otherwise a serious illness, such as polio could result.

Rx

- ✓ Check to be sure all of your children's immunizations are up to date.
- ✓ Insist that your child have a tuberculin skin test yearly or at least every two years.
- ✓ Schedule your child yearly for a complete medical examination by a physician.
- ✓ Have a urinalysis checked yearly.
- ✓ Ask that a blood count be done yearly.
- ✓ Give your child a multi-vitamin daily that is suggested by your doctor, not one from a health food store.
- ✓ Schedule a dental check-up once or twice a year for each child.
- ✓ Insist that each child have a regular bedtime.
- ✓ Have your child eat both breakfast and lunch rather than waiting to eat after school.
- ✓ Ask about any side effects or precautions when a doctor prescribes a medication and ask what it is for.
- ✓ **Don't** give herbal medicines to kids. They can be particularly dangerous for them.
- ✓ Watch that your child doesn't go to the bathroom more than three or four times a day or less often than that; both can be a cause for concern.
- ✓ Give your kids adequate protein, vegetables, and fruits.
- ✓ Insist that your kids drink enough water and not many soft drinks. Too much juice or even excessive milk can be a problem.
- ✓ Have a child who is frequently tired or irritable checked by a physician. Be sure he or she is getting enough sleep.

CONSTIPATION

Julia was brought to my office one Saturday complaining of severe stomach pain. Her parents were worried about appendicitis and this seemed a good possibility. When I examined the little girl, I felt rock hard masses in her tummy and suspected she was just very constipated. An X-ray confirmed this and a child's suppository and an enema relieved the pain. We were all delighted that surgery was not necessary. Marked changes in the child's diet prevented the problem from reoccurring.

Another cute little 3-year-old insisted that "she was not concentrated", when her mother and I were discussing the child's constipation. The mother and I both had a good chuckle about Suzy's choice of words.

Rx

- ✓ Keep a three day record of everything eaten if a child has an on-going problem with constipation.
- ✓ Make sure there is adequate daily protein, fruits, and vegetables.
- ✓ Delete apple sauce and bananas is there is constipation.
- ✓ Give extra water for softer stools.
- ✓ Decrease excessive milk intake if a child is constipated.
- ✓ Watch for a crack or fissure near the anus or rectum. This will make a child hold back bowel movements and cause constipation.
- ✓ Give apricot nectar or prune juice to make stools softer.
- ✓ Be aware that emotional problems can cause a child to hold back bowel movements.
- ✓ Constipation can be present with Celiac disease.

SETTING AN EXAMPLE

A little girl was brought to my office because of difficulties getting along in school. She was angry and hyperactive. I knew the parents were both hardworking and quite intense and sensed that some of the child's behavior was attention getting. I wondered too, if some of her behavior was being modeled on what she saw at home. Kids pick up spoken words; as well as a parent's body language and behavior in public and private. Kids are like sponges and being a parent is a tough, often a no win situation.

Rx

- ✓ Kids quickly learn if a parent is often or always late and constantly rushing.
- ✓ Knowing how to have fun is important for kids to note.
- ✓ If a parent talks more than he or she listens, kids will stop listening.
- ✓ Honking, speeding unnecessarily or parking illegally, as in disabled parking sets a bad example, particularly for new drivers in a family.
- ✓ Swearing will be mimicked by your kids.
- ✓ Lying will set a bad example for your kids when it is discovered.
- ✓ Honesty does pay, particularly with kids.
- ✓ Not making complete stops at stop signs or running red lights will be noted by your kids.
- ✓ Being generally polite and pleasant on the telephone pays off as a parent.
- ✓ Gossiping can set a bad example for kids.
- ✓ Keeping confidences and promises made to kids is important.
- ✓ Valuing things or money more than people will be quickly noted by your children.
- ✓ Writing thank you notes is good role modeling for kids.
- ✓ Having a positive outlook will be noted and appreciated by your children.

TWINS OR MULTIPLE BIRTHS

A mother of twins brought the girls to my office for the first time. One of the twins seemed quite unhappy. After I examined the girls, I asked the nurse to let them play in the waiting room where there were toys and books. In talking with the mother I discovered that the one twin always seemed to take charge and put the other one at a great disadvantage. It seemed that the smaller twin felt she just couldn't compete with her sister and was retreating into her own world. Some play therapy with a children's psychologist helped a great deal and the psychologist helped the parents learn new ways to keep the older twin from taking over.

Rx

- ✓ Always have lots of extra supplies. You'll need them!
- ✓ Treat each twin as a distinct personality.
- ✓ Avoid identical clothes, hairstyles, furniture, or color schemes. Each child needs to have their own identity and not just be half of a whole.
- ✓ Provide playmates now and then for the twins. Twins often want to play just with each other. Many develop their own codes and language and live in their own special world.
- ✓ Place the twins in separate classrooms, if possible when they start school.
- ✓ Join a twin parents' group or find a twin chat-room online.
- ✓ Give other children, if you have them, lots of time and attention.
- ✓ Plan a few minutes time each day just for you. Twins take extra time and energy.
- ✓ Look for each twin's special abilities and encourage these.
- ✓ Try to prevent one twin from always dominating the other.
- ✓ Give each twin equal attention, particularly if one twin has special problems.

CHOOSING HEALTH INSURANCE OR AN HMO

I was an expert witness for the parents in a case where they were suing an obstetrician for malpractice. Their baby had been badly damaged at birth. The court reporter was quite pregnant and when the deposition was over, I asked when her baby was due and where she was delivering. I couldn't believe my ears when she said it was at the same HMO where the doctor, who was being sued, was in practice. It was possible that he would be the one on call when the woman went into labor. I suggested that she needed to look elsewhere for care. The woman said she didn't know how to find a good HMO or know how to decide on which insurance was the best. I sat down with her and made the following suggestions.

Rx

- ✓ Check on the cost of premiums.
- ✓ Find out about any restrictions.
- ✓ Determine what the co-payments will be.
- ✓ Inquire about what surgeries are covered.
- ✓ Find out if prescriptions are covered partly or fully.
- ✓ Check on what hospitalizations are covered and for how many days.
- ✓ Determine if any conditions are excluded from coverage.
- ✓ Inquire about restrictions on outside specialists that can be seen.
- ✓ Read about the appeal process if coverage is denied.
- ✓ Find out how long the HMO has been in business.
- ✓ Determine who owns the HMO.
- ✓ Check on what physicians are included in the HMO or under the insurance.
- ✓ Inquire about what emergencies are covered in other hospitals.

Resources

PARENTING WEBSITES

www.babyzone.com

www.babycenter.com

www.positiveparenting.com

www.parentplace.com

www.parentime.com

www.abcparenting.com

www.fathermag.com

www.parenthoodweb.com

www.parenting.com

www.fathersnetwork.org

www.positiveparenting.com

www.parentplace.com

www.parentime.com

www.parentpals.com (For children with special needs)

www.abcparenting.com

www.brightfutures.org

www.familytravelnetwork.com

www.tripletconnection.org

www.netnanny.com

www.zerotothree.org

www.parent.net

Single Parents

www.singleparentsnet.com

www.singleparentcentral.com

Parents Without Partners

www.parentswithoutpartners.com

Stepfamilies

www.stepfamily.org

www.stepfamilies.com

Healthy Eating

www.healthyeating.net

www.eatright.org

Immunizations

www.cdc.gov

www.immunizationsinfo.org

Health Information

www.kidshealth.org

www.childrenwithdiabetes.com (Information about diabetes)

www.aaaai.org (Information about asthma and allergies)

www.chadd.org (Information about attention deficit disorder)

www.healthfinder.gov

Resources

Consumer Safety
ww.cpsc.org

Adoption
www.adoptivefam.org

www.adoption.org

Missing Kids
www.missingkids.com

Divorce
www.divorcecentral.com

www.divorceonline.com

www.divorceNet.com

www.divorcesupport.com

www.parent.net/parents/resources

For Fathers
www.fathers.com

www.fathersworld.com

www.fathers4kids.org

www.fapt.org

www.fatherhoodproject.org

www.dadsempowered.org

www.stepdads.com

www.divorcefathers.com

Child Care

www.nannycare.com

www.naccrra.net

Recalls

www.recalls.gov

Military Families

www.militarychild.org

MORE RESOURCES

AMERICAN ACADEMY OF PEDIATRICS
141 Northwest Point Blvd.
P. O. Box 927
Elk Village, IL. 60009-0927
1-800-433-9016

NATIONAL CHILD CARE ASSOCIATION
1325 G Street NW
Suite 500
Washington D.C. 20005
1-800-543-7161

NATIONAL HEAD START ASSOCIATION
1651 Prince Street
Alexandria, VA 20003
1-703-739=0875
www.heardstartinfo.org

STEP FAMILY FOUNDATION
310 West 85th Street
Suite 18
New York, NY 10024
1-212-877-3244
or

Resources (151)

1-631-725-0919

COUNCIL ON FAMILY HEALTH
1150 Connecticut Ave.
Suite 1200-B
Washington D.C. 20036
1-08-339-3120

U.S.CONSUMER PRODUCT SAFETY COMMISSION (CPSC)
Washington D.C. 20207
800-638-2772
www.cpsc.gov
(Send a postcard to ask for the Child Care Safety Checklist)

HELPFUL VIDEOS

BABY AND CHILD CPR

Child CPR Training — www.procpr.org

ABDUCTION

KidSmartz-an information video on prevention of abduction
www.imdb.com/title/tt0re5103/

HELPFUL 800 NUMBERS

Lactation Hotline	877-452-5324
La Leche League	800-525-3243
National CDC Information Hotline	800-232-2522
Nanny Care	800-383-5136
Au Pair in America	800-928-7247
Child Care Association	800-543-7161
Consumer Product Safety	800-638-2772
National Resources for Disabilities	800-644-2666

Parental Stress Line	800-632-8188
National Easter Seal Society	800-221-6827
National Center for Stuttering	800-221-2483
National Health Information	800-336-4797
U.S. Consumer Product Safety Commission	800-638-2772
National Mental Health Association Help Line	800-969-6642
National Center for Learning Disabilities	800-575-7373
Childhelp USA	800-422-4435
Child Abuse Hotline	800-422-4453
National Adoption Center	800-862-3678
National Child Care Association	800-543-7161
Child Care Aware	800-424-2246
Parents Without Partners	800-637-7974
National Health Information Center Referral Service	800-336-4797
National Down Syndrome Society	800-221-4602
American Speech-Language-Hearing Association	800-638-8255
Juvenile Diabetes Foundation	800-223-1138
Step Family Association of America	800-735-0329
Association for Marriage and Family Therapy	800-374-2638
United Cerebral Palsy	800-872-1827
Child Find of America	800-426-5678
Child Care Aware	800-424-2246
Poison Control Center	800-222-1222
Safety Belt Safe U.S.A.	800-745-SAFE
Growing Child	800-927-7289

Bibliography

Adams, Jerry. How to Raise Disciplined and Happy Children. CreateSpace, Charleston, S.C. 2011.

Brott, Armin. *The New Father: A Dad's Guide to the Toddler Years.* Abbeville Press, New York, NY 2004.

Conner, Bobbi, G*uide to Raising Great Kids.* Bantam Books, New York, NY 1997.

Conner, Bobbi. *Everyday Opportunities for Extraordinary Parenting.* Sourcebooks, Naperville, IL 2000.

Conner, Bobbi. *The Giant Book of Creativity for Kids.* Roost Books, Boston, MA, 2015.

Crary, Elizabeth. *365 Wacky Wonderful Ways to Get Kids to Do What You Want.*

Parenting Press, Seattle, WA, 1995.

Ferro, Pamela. *The Everything Twins, Triplets and More.* Adams Media, Avon, MA. 2005.

Greenberg, Gary, Jeannie Hayden. *A Practical Handbooks for New Dads.* Simon and Schuster, New York, NY 2004.

Koman, Aleta and Myers, Edward. *The Parenting Survival Kit.* Perigee Trade, New York, NY, 2000.

Katz, Adrienne. *What to do with Kids on a Rainy Day or in a Car, on a Train or When They are Sick.* St. Martin's Press, New York, NY, 1989

Leach, Penelope. *Your Baby and Child: From Birth to Age Five,* Knopf. New York, NY, 2010.

Linden, Dana, Emma Paroli, Mia Aoron, *Preemies.* Pocket Books, New York, NY 2000.

Moskwinski, Rebecca. *Twins to Quints: The Complete Manual for Parents of Multiple Birth Children.* Brentwood, TN. 2002.

Spock, Benjamin and Robert Needman. Dr. Spock's Baby and Child Care. Gallery Books, New York, NY, 2012.

Thompson, Charlotte. *Raising a Handicapped Child.* Oxford University Press, New York, NY 1999.

Thompson, Charlotte. *Raising a Child with a Neuromuscular Disorder.* Oxford University Press, New York, NY, 2000.

Thompson, Charlotte. *101 Ways To The Best Medical Care.* Infinity Publishers, Conshohocken, PA 2006.

Whitlock, Natalie. *A Parent's Guide to the Internet.* Mars Publishing Inc, Minneapolis, MN, 2003.

Warner, Penny. *Healthy Snacks for Kids.* Nitty Gritty Cookbooks, Concord, CA, 2007.

Index

A
Anemia, 46, 48, 53, 102

B
Bottle, 9, 11, 14, 15, 22, 53, 133

Breast pump, 9

C
Christening, 31

Cornstarch, 29

D
Deaf, 82

Diarrhea, 9, 23, 99, 120, 131

E
Educational psychologist, 49, 51, 75, 103, 126, 134, 139

F
Fathers' group, 13

G
Gymboree, 16

J
Jaundice, 18

L
La Leche League, 16, 151

N

New mothers' group, 12

P

Post-partum depression, 13

Pus, 18, 60

R

Rectal thermometer, 23, 37

Rice cereal, 36

S

SIDS, 36

Soap, 29, 44

T

Teething rings, 32

Thyroid, 17, 18

W

Weight gain, 17, 18, 46